Neuroscience, Psychology, *and* Religion

Templeton Science and Religion Series

In our fast-paced and high-tech era, when visual information seems so dominant, the need for short and compelling books has increased. This conciseness and convenience is the goal of the Templeton Science and Religion Series. We have commissioned scientists in a range of fields to distill their experience and knowledge into a brief tour of their specialties. They are writing for a general audience, readers with interests in the sciences or the humanities, which includes religion and theology. The relationship between science and religion has been likened to four types of doorways. The first two enter a realm of "conflict" or "separation" between these two views of life and the world. The next two doorways, however, open to a world of "interaction" or "harmony" between science and religion. We have asked our authors to enter these latter doorways to judge the possibilities. They begin with their sciences and, in aiming to address religion, return with a wide variety of critical viewpoints. We hope these short books open intellectual doors of every kind to readers of all backgrounds.

Series Editors: J. Wentzel van Huyssteen & Khalil Chamcham
Project Editor : Larry Witham

Neuroscience, Psychology, *and* Religion

ILLUSIONS, DELUSIONS, AND REALITIES
ABOUT HUMAN NATURE

Malcolm Jeeves and Warren S. Brown

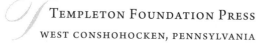

TEMPLETON FOUNDATION PRESS
WEST CONSHOHOCKEN, PENNSYLVANIA

Templeton Foundation Press
300 Conshohocken State Road, Suite 550
West Conshohocken, PA 19428
www.templetonpress.org

Designed and typeset by Gopa &Ted2, Inc.

Templeton Foundation Press helps intellectual leaders and others learn about science research on aspects of realities, invisible and intangible. Spiritual realities include unlimited love, accelerating creativity, worship, and the benefits of purpose in persons and in the cosmos.

Library of Congress Cataloging-in-Publication Data
Jeeves, Malcolm A., 1926–
  Neuroscience, psychology, and religion / Malcolm Jeeves and
Warren S. Brown.
     p. cm.
  Includes bibliographical references and index.
  ISBN-13: 978-1-59947-147-1 (alk. paper)
  ISBN-10: 1-59947-147-7 (alk. paper)
  1. Psychology and religion. 2. Psychology, Religious. 3. Neurosciences.
4. Religion. I. Brown, Warren S., 1944- II. Title.
  BL53.J5 2009
  201'.615—dc22
                                                    2008031787

Printed in the United States of America

09 10 11 12 13 14   10 9 8 7 6 5 4 3 2 1

Contents

Preface

AT TIMES, science develops very fast. Neuroscience and psychology are in one of those periods, with research at the interface of these fields moving at a breathless pace. We have progressed from the "Decade of the Brain" in the 1990s, to the "Decade of the Mind" at the beginning of the twenty-first century. It seems as though we are now looking forward to the "Decade of the Mind/Brain." All this development has been fueled by new research technologies, notably developments in brain-imaging techniques. The result: no area of our existence seems safe from the probing eyes of the brain scanners. Even our religious experiences have come within the scrutiny of "neurotheologists." The research findings seem so critical to the understanding of our selves as human beings that they are frequently given wide publicity outside of the academy.

What are we to make of it all? How much of our understanding of human nature are we being called upon to rethink? Do we have a soul? Are we apes on the way up or angels on the way down? Is the human mind, including religion and religious experiences, to be reduced to nothing other than the outcome of the rules governing the functioning of neurons and their molecular structures?

This book attempts to help you, the reader, gain understanding and perspective on what is currently happening in research in neuroscience and psychology. Throughout these chapters, you will encounter thought-provoking material, such as descriptions of brain systems and processes involved in the most sophisticated aspects of mental life and comparisons of the neuropsychology of humans and nonhuman primates. You will also find accounts of studies of brain function and religious beliefs and experiences. In all of these areas of research, we have attempted to provide you with relevant contexts and perspectives—historical, philosophical, and theological—for rethinking your concepts of human nature.

Neuropsychology is a specialist scientific field that works at the junction between neuroscience and psychology. We are both neuropsychologists. We also share a common research interest in parts of the brain that connect the two cerebral hemispheres, primarily the corpus callosum. One of us, Warren Brown, continues actively researching in this area (at the Fuller Graduate School of Psychology in California), working with collaborators at California Institute of Technology, University of California San Francisco, and Brigham Young University. The other, Malcolm Jeeves, though supposedly retired, continues to interact with scientists and laboratories with international reputations in both neuroscience and evolutionary psychology (at the University of St. Andrews in Scotland).

As well as enthusiastic scientists, we are also both active Christians, sharing the challenges that scientific discoveries pose for some traditional Christian beliefs. In what follows, we invite you to look at our responses to some of these challenges, see where we have got to in our thinking, and decide what you make of it all.

At the end, we give an extensive index and a list of further reading for those who may wish to follow up in greater depth some of the ideas raised by what we have written. We hope you enjoy reading it as much as we have writing it.

Neuroscience, Psychology, *and* Religion

CHAPTER 1
Neuroscience and Psychology Today

THE ISSUES of neuroscience arise every day in our modern world. We hear about the sad effects of Alzheimer's disease on the elderly but also those stories of patients waking from comas, regaining their ability to speak—as if nothing had happened. Soldiers return from the battlefield suffering from brain damage they received in combat. Our Western literature also gives occasional glimpses of what happens when the workings of the brain go wrong, and perhaps none is more memorable than the account given by the Russian writer Fyodor Dostoyevsky in his novel *The Idiot*. In this story, the character Prince Myshkin has bouts of epilepsy. During a brief "pause" before a seizure begins, he notices that

> his brain was on fire, and in an extraordinary surge all his vital forces would be intensified. The sense of life, the consciousness of self, were multiplied tenfold in these moments. . . . His mind and heart were flooded with extraordinary light; all torment, all doubt, all anxieties were relieved at once, resolved in a kind of lofty calm, full of serene, harmonious joy and hope, full of understanding and the knowledge of the ultimate cause of things. . . . If in that second—that is, in the last lucid moment before the fit—he had time to say to himself clearly and consciously: "Yes, one might give one's whole life for this moment!" then that moment by itself would certainly be worth the whole of life.[1]

Although this is literary fiction, the description accords well with the extensive literature showing how unusual religious experiences are sometimes associated with temporal lobe seizures. Dostoyevsky himself had epilepsy, and this passage may well describe his own seizure experiences.

This book introduces readers to the wide range of issues in modern neuroscience and psychology, but it will take a particular interest in the topic raised by Dostoyevsky's compelling account: the role of brain activity in human behavior, experience, and even religious belief. Given the clear relationship between brain activity (abnormal activity, in this case) and its manifestations in psychological and religious subjective experiences, how should we view human experiences? Are human behavior and experience nothing more than the outcome of the physiological functioning of neurons or of the laws of physical chemistry governing the molecules that make up neurons? This consideration finally leads us to the specific question of how human nature can be interpreted from the perspectives of science, religious worldviews, and our inner subjective experiences.

In the past few decades, developments at the interface of psychology and neuroscience have seen remarkable advances. Psychology has also been hitting the headlines where it interfaces with evolutionary biology, generating the new specialty of evolutionary psychology. As the headlines also attest, some scientists have interpreted this progress as a confirmation of atheism—that is, if important properties of human nature, such as religiousness, can be shown to be aspects of the natural world, then any religious view must be ruled out. Both the popular science writer Richard Dawkins and Nobel laureate Francis Crick have published widely read books arguing this point. Crick spelled out what he saw as some of the radical implications of developments in neuroscience in his book *The Astonishing Hypothesis* (1994).

This debate is not new, of course. Throughout the history and development of psychology and neuroscience, leading figures have written about the implications of this research for traditional religious beliefs. Some have written as theists and others as atheists. Leading figures in psychology who were theists include William James, Carl Jung, Gordon Allport, and Sir Frederic Bartlett. Among the atheists are Sigmund Freud and B. F. Skinner. In neuroscience, a leading theist was Sir John Eccles and a leading atheist Francis Crick, both Nobel laureates. When we see such distinguished scientists in psychology and neuroscience taking these radically different views on religion, the lesson becomes clear: there are no easy answers to these questions. There are no knockdown arguments to settle the debates. In these pages, we will explore the dialogue between a religious worldview and the rapidly accumulating new results from human neuroscience and psychology.

Neuroscience

For the past half century, the field of neuroscience has experienced remarkable growth, from an undesignated scattering of research enterprises to one of the largest, fastest-growing, and most rapidly advancing fields of science. The commitment of both the scientific community and governments to research in neuroscience was underlined in the minds of the public when the U.S. Congress declared the last ten years of the twentieth century "The Decade of the Brain." The consequence of this was a significant increase in research funding for neuroscience. This rapid growth is also reflected in the increase in the number of active researchers in neuroscience over the past thirty years. At the inaugural meeting of the Society for Neuroscience in 1969, there were a hundred participants. In 2005, there were more than thirty thousand. In the same year, leaders of nine nations within the European Community became sufficiently concerned about the wider implications of research in psychology and neuroscience that they set up a commission to report on these. [2]

New technologies have fueled this rapid growth of research. The most important advance is a new means of imaging the human brain in a nonintrusive manner—that is, in a manner akin to taking a simple x-ray. Magnetic resonance imaging (MRI) allows scientists to look at the structure and integrity of brain tissue inside the skull of a patient or research participant. Then, using *functional* MRI (fMRI), it is possible to superimpose on the MRI's brain image an additional representation of areas that are relatively more metabolically active. By this, patterns of brain activity can be observed during a particular mental state or while accomplishing a cognitive task. For example, brain activity can be seen in the language areas of the left cerebral cortex when a person is asked to provide verbs to accompany nouns. Another research tool, positron emission tomography (PET), is very much like fMRI in providing information about the distribution of mental activity in the brain. These are the most often used of an increasingly large array of brain-imaging techniques that are still being developed.

New technologies are also allowing scientists to refine older methods of studying the brain in living subjects. Prior to the advent of brain imaging, neuroscience had focused on experimental studies of animals or relied on the clinical observations and behaviors of people with brain damage or brain disease. Now there is a way to experiment harmlessly with such interruptions to the brain. This is possible with transcranial magnetic stimulation, a technology that gives scientists a reversible method of temporarily disrupting brain activity in selective areas. Thus, research on the effects of the disruption of function is no longer limited to experimentally damaging (or stimulating) brain areas in animals or to studying accidental damage in humans.

With the tools of imaging, neuroscience has also begun to tackle the highest forms of human cognitive and social functioning. For example, researchers have imaged brain activity while a person is involved in moral reasoning or while experiencing empathy for another human being—a topic we will review in later chapters.

PSYCHOLOGY

The term *psychology* comes from a Greek word referring to the mind. In the early years, psychologists agreed that their field was principally about the internal processes of a human mind under study. However, frustrated by the fact that minds of other people cannot be studied directly, psychological science shifted dramatically to experiments and theories only about people's behavior. This shift took place by the middle of the twentieth century (in a movement led by B. F. Skinner). In this view, behavior was all that existed. Any talk of mind was, at best, unscientific. This was the era of behaviorism. But the pendulum has swung back. Since the last quarter of the twentieth century, psychology has moved in a direction heralded now as the "cognitive revolution." Theories about inner mental states (consciousness, emotion, memory, etc.) have all been allowed back into the field.

The contemporary move to neuroscience research has also occurred among many psychologists, but it took longer in their profession. Either way, the field has grown dramatically. When the American Psychological Association was founded in 1892, there were 131 members, associate members, and fellows. When it divided into the American Psychological Association and the American Psychological Society in 1988, there were 66,996 affiliates.

The field of psychology is broad in its subject matter. Scan the contents of a contemporary college textbook of psychology and you understand why it is so difficult to pigeonhole psychology as a biological science or a behavioral science or a social science. However, most today would agree that large parts of contemporary psychology can quite properly be labeled as scientific.

It has been more than a century since William James wrote to his friend Thomas W. Ward, "It seems to me that perhaps the time has come for psychology to be a science."[3] Psychologist Howard Gardner, like James a professor at Harvard, was still reflecting on this issue in his 1988 William James Lecture entitled, "Scientific

Psychology: Should We Bury It or Praise It?" Gardner believed that "psychology has not added up to an integrated science, and it is unlikely ever to achieve that status." He continued:

> What does make sense is to recognize important insights that have been achieved by psychologists; to identify the contribution which contemporary psychology can make to disciplines which may someday achieve a firmer scientific status; and finally to determine whether these parts of psychology might survive as participants in the conversation which obtains across major disciplines.[4]

As an aside he added, "For the most part, psychologists (like other academics) go about their daily research and writing without agonizing about the actual or potential coherence of their field."[5] Most psychologists are content to accept as their primary goal to produce "reliable knowledge."

While debate about the scientific status of some areas of psychology will no doubt continue, most agree that, in the case of *neuropsychology*—which is where psychology interfaces with neuroscience—there is no doubt about its scientific status. This area of psychology will be the focus of this book as we consider the science's impact on religion and religious beliefs.

RELATING SCIENCE AND RELIGION

Throughout the last century, it became increasingly clear that both psychology and neuroscience pose difficult questions for the religious views of most people. The liveliest debates have occurred in two fast-developing fields. The first is neuropsychology, the study of the neurological basis of human thought and behavior. And the second is evolutionary psychology, the study of the likely evolutionary emergence of human thought and behavior. It is fair to say that the scientific status of these two areas of contemporary psychology is widely accepted. Although they may be regarded as part of "the scientific enterprise," that phrase itself has been used in a variety of different ways over the past four centuries. Moreover, we seem to be continuing that long, historical debate on how exactly to relate this accumulating "scientific" knowledge to traditional theological statements.

Most scholars agree that, by the seventeenth century, Puritan scientists, such as John Wallis, William Petty, William Turner, Henry Briggs, John Bainbridge, and John Wilkins (many of whom were founding members of the Royal Society of London), regarded science as an ally of true religion. In a spirit of optimism today, we might even admire the protagonists of "free science" among the Puritans (who otherwise held revelation as their highest authority). Wary of mere human authority, they pitted their free science—which was "not adorned by great names but naked and simple"—against what they regarded as the superstitious cult of Aristotle. For Puritans, it was not freedom that led to truth, but truth that led to freedom.[6]

For those who had stood on Aristotle's teaching, it was only "natural" and "reasonable" to move from his idea of living things as embodiments of eternal forms or unchanging essences to the idea of species as fixed and unchanging. Eventually, the evolutionary ideas of Charles Darwin shook this Aristotelian biology at its very foundation. What if species are not fixed? What if there is a measure of change from generation to generation? What Newton had done to Aristotelian physics, Darwin did to Aristotelian biology. With this challenge Darwin, like Newton, produced a point of departure for a new worldview. Newton's intelligently designed machine would, under Darwin's influence, acquire the properties of a dynamic and progressive organism.

Some may find it strange that aspects of Darwin's views of humankind had simply recaptured the Hebrew–Christian emphasis on human beings as a part of nature. Nature, said Darwin, includes both man and his culture. By contrast, the Greek tendency was to separate humankind from the rest of creation and to give human beings and human minds an arrogant, aristocratic place over nature. Darwin's views also challenged any simple analogy of God as the "maker" of the universe—that is, as an absentee landlord who made the world and then left it to run autonomously. But historical puzzles remain. Given that Hebrew–Christian thinking about nature encouraged the rise of science and that Christian thinkers developed scientific research, why do we now say that science and religion are in conflict? This topic has been dealt with at length by several scholars.[7] They have traced out the origins and recurrence of the "warfare metaphor." Although "warfare" readily describes debates over creation and evolution, it also remains near the surface in debates about scientific and biblical views of human nature. Neuropsychology and evolutionary psychology have produced much of our best scientific data on human nature, and so, unfortunately, these are fertile fields for the new advocates of "warfare" between science and religion.

By the end of this book, readers will have a greater sense of the puzzles that neuroscience and psychology have produced in regard to human nature and the religious nature of humankind. We begin our journey in chapter 2 by laying out the two perennial options—warfare or partnership—in the relationship between brain science and religion. We will show in chapter 3, however, that some of these issues are not as new as is claimed. Next, we move to the physical functioning of the brain: chapter 4 presents a model of brain activity that is helpful when interpreting claims about the physical nature of psychological and religious experience; and chapter 5 shows how tightly bound—or "embodied"—mental activity is with the brain's physical activity.

As we approach the question of human nature, we must look at our evolutionary history and our relationship to nonhuman primate cousins—the topic of chapter 6. In chapter 7, we return to the type of questions raised by Dostoyevsky's novel: how are scientists tying religious experience to particular events of the brain, such as temporal lobe seizures, or to particular "spots" in the brain?

All of these findings have an impact on a central concept in Western thought, that of human beings in the "image of God." So chapter 8 will survey the new ways of interpreting this concept. We conclude in chapter 9 with a synthesis of neuroscience, psychology, and religion—that we shall generally call *emergent*—that we feel is a compelling solution for our modern understanding.

CHAPTER 2
Warfare versus Partnership

ENORMOUS STRIDES are being made in research in both neuroscience and psychology. But with each new discovery, partisans have seized on the latest findings as weaponry in the ongoing, and at times contentious, debate between science and religion. Now as in the past, we invariably meet the outspoken voices on both sides of this debate: some say brain science and religion are in a perennial battle, while others claim that a constructive partnership can be forged.

There are science-minded and religious-minded people on both sides of this debate. Among the proponents of "warfare," some scientists argue that scientific information trumps all religious views, while religious voices often respond by rejecting all scientific theory as a rival to traditional religious commitments. On the other hand, there are many who would argue (including the authors of this volume) that, with appropriate adjustments and open reflection on both sides, there is the real possibility of a partnership between scientific and religious views of humankind.

This dynamic holds especially true for the psychological sciences and religion. The "warfare" metaphor has often been popular, as it continues to be in our own day. It is not unusual to hear highly intelligent and well-informed people repeat the claim that psychology in general, and Sigmund Freud in particular, have "explained away" religious beliefs as "nothing but" wishful thinking; they say it is merely whistling in the dark of an empty universe, hoping to keep up our spirits. In this sense, the warfare metaphor is alive and well as a shorthand in the twenty-first century.

In most centuries, some variation of the warfare theme has been used. Some have argued, for example, that "warfare" best characterized the relationship between science and religion in the nineteenth century. Historians of science have been discrediting this idea, however, as seen in the work of Laurence Hearnshaw.[1] He identified four significant influences—what we might call a trend toward a science-religion "partnership"—at the end of the nineteenth century that provided the basis for later psychological studies of religion:

1. studies of the manifestations of religion, as in British geneticist Francis Galton's study of prayer
2. studies by anthropologists of comparative religion and the origins of religion, typified by Scottish anthropologist Sir James Fraser
3. the writings of theologians on mysticism and religious experiences, such as that of the Anglican clergyman William R. Inge
4. the beginnings of the systematic psychology of religion, as done by psychologist Edwin G. Starbuck.

These trends culminated in Harvard psychologist William James' classic *The Varieties of Religious Experience* (1902). It is noteworthy that none of the authors listed above seems to have been motivated by a desire to generate or perpetuate a warfare metaphor to describe the relationship between psychology and religion. Certainly, in the case of James, the relationship was clearly a strongly positive one as he sought to explore how psychology could deepen our understanding of the roots and fruits of religion.

As we move into the twentieth century, the picture changes so that, by the time Freud's radical views were becoming more widely known in society, the stage was set for a strong resurgence of the warfare metaphor. A closer look shows that Freud never said that his accounts of religious origins passed judgment on the truth-value of specific beliefs; he said this must be decided on other grounds. Nevertheless, Freud was generally seen as "explaining away" religious beliefs and arguing that religious practice was "nothing but" a social neurosis to be grown out of.

In due course, Freud's views on the origins of religion in *Totem and Taboo* (1919) and *Moses and Monotheism* (1938) were severely criticized, as many of the so-called facts on which he based his theories were shown by professional anthropologists to be incorrect. This did little in the popular mind, however, to bring Freud's views into disrespect.[2] Freud had produced a good story, and his influence in this, as in other areas, persisted long after his views were widely discredited by scholars in related disciplines.

Much the same may be said about Freud's views of religion in *The Future of an Illusion* (1927) and *Civilization and Its Discontents* (1930). In Freud's terminology, an "illusion" stands for any belief system based on human wishes. He was careful to point out that such a basis does not necessarily imply that the system is false; nevertheless, as far as Christianity was concerned, he clearly believed that it was. In that sense, he championed and perpetuated a form of warfare between psychology and religion.

Another major figure in psychology during the first half of the twentieth century was Carl Jung. For a time, Jung was a close collaborator with Freud, though he subsequently developed his own views within the psychoanalytic tradition. Freud and Jung, as in matters psychological, ultimately differed radically in their views of religion. Whereas Freud said religion was a neurosis that must be dispelled to cure the patient (that is, the human race), Jung viewed religion as an essential human activity. The task of psychology was not to explain away religion but to try to understand how human nature reacts to situations normally described as religious.

Freud's and Jung's contrasting views were aptly summarized by G. S. Spinks:

> For Freud religion was an obsessional neurosis, and at no time did he modify that judgment. For Jung it was the absence of religion that was the chief cause of adult psy-

chological disorders. These two sentences indicate how great the difference is between their respective stand points on religion.[3]

Freud and Jung captured the headlines and the public interest in what was happening at the psychology–religion interface of their day. But there were others, such as Robert Thouless, who were writing on the same topic. In the view of many psychologists, Thouless made a far more lasting contribution. His 1930s book, *Introduction to the Psychology of Religion*, was reprinted as late as 1971 for continued use. Thouless' approach was primarily constructive and in stark contrast to the warfare metaphor.

Since World War II, there have been several noteworthy attempts to offer new insights into religion through the eyes of psychology. Notable among these are Gordon Allport's *The Individual and His Religion* (1951), and Michael Argyle's several books, including *Religious Behavior* (1958) (with Beit Hallahmi) and *The Social Psychology of Religion* (1975). These, like Thouless' book, are not confrontational and bear no mark of the warfare approach. These works are read by psychologists and others interested in deepening their understanding of psychology and religion. Lacking confrontation, these books do not stir uproars or publicity. Such, however, was not the case with B. F. Skinner's views of religion.

Skinner's views were perhaps the most widely publicized of the warfare genre in the second half of the twentieth century because of his well-deserved reputation as the leading behaviorist psychologist of this era. Having achieved considerable success in the development of techniques for shaping and modifying behavior, Skinner went on to speculate about how such techniques might be harnessed to shape the future of society. He believed that principles of rewards and punishments could even explain how the practice of religion functions psychologically. "The religious agency," he said, "is a special form of government under which 'good' and 'bad' become 'pious' and 'sinful.' Contingencies involving positive and negative reinforcement, often of the most extreme sort, are codified—for example as commandments, maintained by specialists, usually with the support of ceremonies, rituals and stories."[4] He argued that the good things, personified in a god, are reinforcing, whereas the threat of hell is an aversive stimulus. Both are used to shape behavior.

Underlying Skinner's approach is a reductionist presupposition. He speaks of concepts of god being "reduced to" what we find positively reinforcing. There is no doubt that Skinner provided ready ammunition for anyone wishing to perpetuate the warfare metaphor in psychology and religion.

While Skinner became the champion of this metaphor, he was counterbalanced by another great psychologist of that period: Roger Sperry. A psychologist, neuroscientist and Nobel Laureate, Sperry wrote that some forms of behaviorism were bankrupt. Behaviorism did not hold up in the face of the new cognitive sciences, which gave thinking and consciousness a central role in behavior. Thus, Sperry advocated the benefits of a positive relationship between psychology and religion. He viewed them as allies engaged in a common task. We must note, however, that Sperry's views of religion would sound strange to ordinary religious individuals. Typical of Sperry's views is the following:

> The answer to the question, "Is there convergence between science and religion?" seems from the standpoint of psychology to be a definite emphatic "yes." Over the past fifteen years, changes in the foundational concepts of psychology instituted by the new cognitive or mentalist paradigm have radically reformed scientific descriptions of human nature, and the conscious self. The resultant views are today less atomistic, less mechanistic, and more mentalistic, contextual, subjectivistic and humanistic. From the standpoint of theology, these new mentalistic tenets, which no longer exclude on princi-

ple the entire inner world of subjective phenomena, are much more palatable and compatible than were those of the behaviorist-materialist era. Where science and religion had formerly stood in direct conflict on this matter to the point even of being mutually exclusive and irreconcilable, one now sees a new compatibility, potentially even harmony with liberal religion—defined as religion that does not rely on dualistic or supernatural beliefs, forms of which have been increasingly evident in contemporary theology.[5]

From the above quote, several things are clear. Although Sperry had once used the warfare metaphor to characterize science and religion, he felt that psychology had now moved beyond that. Psychology no longer reduced human behavior to nothing but reinforced habits. It now credited the power of subjective experience, thought, and will—and this allowed a more open and compatible relation between religion and psychology. Needless to say, Sperry placed his hopes in a liberal theology that makes no supernatural claims. Hence, we don't think that traditional religious beliefs can readily embrace Sperry's views. His theological views bear little relationship to those of most religious people, and yet what he has written remains worthy of careful consideration.

FROM "WARFARE" TO PARTNERSHIP

The warming trend between science and religion is always beset by the lingering belief that psychology has somehow "explained away" religion. So it is helpful, once again, to look at leading psychologists who have taken the partnership approach. Two noteworthy examples are Gordon Allport in the United States and Sir Frederic Bartlett in Great Britain. They both emphasized the potential for psychology to be positive and sympathetic toward religion. Significantly, they also underscored the limits of psychological inquiry, at least when practiced as a science. Allport, a major influence on the development of theories of personality, wrote:

> [D]ifferent as are science and art in their axioms and methods, they have learned to cooperate in a thousand ways—in the production of fine dwellings, music, clothing, design. Why should not science and religion, likewise differing in axioms and method, yet cooperate in the production of an improved human character without which all other human gains are tragic loss? From many sides today comes the demand that religion and psychology busy themselves in finding a common ground for uniting their efforts for human welfare.[6]

Bartlett, often described as one of the precursors and architects of "the cognitive revolution" in psychology, wrote:

> It is inevitable that the forms which are taken by feeling, thinking, and action within any religion should be molded and directed by the character of its own associated culture. The psychologist must accept these forms and attempt to show how they have grown up and what are their principal effects. Should he appear to succeed in doing these things, he is tempted to suppose that this confers upon him some special right to pronounce upon the further and deeper issues of ultimate truth and value. These issues, as many people have claimed, seem to be inevitably bound up with the assertion that in some way the truth and the worth of religion come from a contact of the natural order with some other order or world, not itself directly accessible to the common human senses. So far as any final decision upon the validity or value of such a claim goes, the psychologist is in exactly the same position as that of any other human being who cares to

consider the matter seriously. Being a psychologist gives him neither superior nor inferior authority.[7]

Both Allport and Bartlett held a high view of the potential benefits of the developing science of psychology. They recognized the distinctive approach to the gaining of knowledge that is made possible through the scientific enterprise—a view already well articulated by leading physical scientists of earlier generations. As should be clear, the secular field of psychology had a mixture of views on the relationship of science and religion. But the purveyors of the "warfare" theme were not always the secular critics of religion. Some Christians were just as antagonistic toward psychology. According to psychologist Hendrika Vande Kemp,

> the antipsychologists seem to regard psychology as offering alternative answers to the same questions answered by Christian theology and biblical revelation, questions concerning knowledge of God and salvation history and a proper human response to both. Psychologists, for the most part, are not interested in "knowing God." They are interested in what kinds of images of God persons entertain and what beliefs they embrace, and how their faith relates to practice—but these involve "knowledge" of a very different sort.[8]

NEUROPSYCHOLOGY
AND EVOLUTIONARY PSYCHOLOGY

Currently we are witnessing a rebirth of Freud's labeling of religious belief as "the future of an illusion" in the widely publicized description by Richard Dawkins of religion as "the God delusion." And Dawkins is not alone. He has ready allies in, for example, the philosopher Daniel Dennett. Dawkins has no doubt that religion is nothing more than a useless, and sometimes dangerous, evolutionary accident. He writes, "Religious behavior may be a misfiring, an unfortunate by-product of an underlying psychological propensity which in other circumstances is, or once was, useful."[9]

Dawkins' views are not universally held, even among evolutionary psychologists. In fact, there is another debate taking place, not between science and religion but within science itself—among scientists studying the evolution of religion. Whereas they agree that religious belief is an outgrowth of brain architecture that evolved during early human history, they disagree about why this tendency to believe evolved at all. Was it because belief itself is adaptive? Or was it because it was just an evolutionary by-product, the mere consequence of some other evolutionary adaptation of the human brain? In sum, do we believe because of an evolutionary neurological accident or because of evolutionary adaptation?

The evolutionary view of human psychology has caused some people to wonder whether we are hardwired to believe in God. Those who follow this track draw upon recent results from brain imaging that seem to locate a "God spot" within the brain—that is, a place in the brain that is active only during religious experiences. Although the idea of a "God spot" may be new, the idea of an organic basis for our beliefs is certainly not. More than a hundred years ago William James, in his *Varieties of Religious Experience*, wrote, "All of our raptures and our drynesses, our longings and pantings, our questions and beliefs . . . are equally organically founded."[10]

This contemporary debate on whether belief evolved as a by-product or as an adaptation reveals that adherents on all sides do not fall neatly into religious and nonreligious outlooks. As you watch the debate, you might expect that only unbelievers adopt the by-product viewpoint, since they want to explain religion as "just a fluke." You might also expect that religious thinkers will always take the adaptation view, since it supports the providential idea of nature's providing emotional, spiritual, and other advantages that accompany faith. But you would be wrong. In each case, the personal religious views of the scientists do not predict which side they are on. As we mentioned above, these issues are complex. There are no simple answers. The positions taken by various persons can sometimes be surprising.

One of the by-product theorists, for example, is American psychologist Justin Barrett at Oxford University. Some of his views resonate with those of evolutionary biologist Stephen Jay Gould, who saw religion as what he described as a "spandrel." Together with his Harvard colleague, geneticist Richard Lewontin, Gould proposed that traits that arise and have no adaptive value of their own should be regarded as spandrels. They borrowed the term from architecture, where it originally referred to the V-shaped structure formed between two rounded arches. The structure is not there for any purpose; it is there because that is what happens when arches align. In architecture, a spandrel can be neutral or it can be made functional—either way it is an unintended by-product. Gould wrote, "Natural selection made the human brain big but most of our mental properties and potentials may be spandrels—that is nonadaptive consequences of building a device with such structural complexity."[11]

It is further argued that some of the hardships of early human life favor the evolution of specific cognitive abilities. Among these was the ability to infer, or detect, the presence of an organism that might do us harm (the proverbial snake rustling the grass or a creaking in the woods). These realities prompted the mind to evolve a "causal narrative" for natural events, eventually leading to the conclusion that other people also have minds of their own. Early human thinking eventually operated on the belief that things in nature have causes and, more specifically, that other people also have minds that contain beliefs, desires, and intentions. Psychologists have variously labeled these evolved mental abilities as *agent detection, causal reasoning,* and *theory of mind.*

For thinkers such as Barrett, who is a Christian, these evolutionary findings simply mean that our brains are primed for religious belief, ready to presume the presence of agents even when such presence confounds logic. "The most central concepts in religions are related to agents," he writes. While it might seem that evolutionary psychology would demand skepticism to supernatural reality, Barrett responds by saying, "Christian theology teaches that people were crafted by God to be in a loving relationship with him and other people. Why wouldn't God, then, design us in such a way as to find belief in divinity quite natural?" Because we have a scientific explanation for a mental phenomenon, he argues, that does not require the end of belief in reality beyond. He asks, for example, "Suppose science produces a convincing account for why I think my wife loves me—should I then stop believing that she does?"[12]

"Nothing Buttery"

We have already noted the ever-present temptation to believe that scientific descriptions can reduce human life, including religion, to nothing more than biological or physical processes. Despite his disclaimers, Francis Crick, in his book *The Astonishing Hypothesis*, reveals a commitment to such "nothing buttery," writing, "You are no more than the behavior of a vast assembly of nerve cells and their associated molecules. . . . You are nothing but a pack of neurons." But the logical conclusion to Crick's argument would be that his own written words about his "astonishing hypothesis" are nothing but ink strokes, carrying no message. Even he drew back at the end, saying, "The words 'nothing but' in our hypothesis can be misleading if understood in too naive a way."[13] As his fellow Nobel laureate Roger Sperry wrote, "The meaning of the message will not be found in the chemistry of the ink."[14]

Similarly, we have seen that Skinner described religious behavior and ideas of God as the product of conditioning, thus "explaining away" religion by reducing it to simple positive reinforcement. This is tantamount to saying that a "no smoking" sign is "nothing but" ink on paper and, therefore, it is perfectly acceptable to go on smoking. Or it is like saying that, when a computer solves a mathematical equation, it is "nothing but" electronics. Mathematicians operating the computer believe they are solving a mathematical equation. They would find it odd to hear that they are merely "making translations" of electronic processes set up by the hardware engineers.

In later pages, as we write about psychology and neuroscience, our enthusiasm for both of these disciplines will be evident. No doubt some of the things that we believe today will be out of date within a decade, so rapidly is the science developing. However, we are, and can continue to be, enthusiastic about our science and without distress regarding new and surprising discoveries that might give challenging new insights into the remarkable complexity of our human nature. We neither remain in a state of constant anxiety lest the latest discovery will "explain away" some of our religious beliefs nor reduce them to "nothing but" physics or chemistry. To paraphrase Sperry's comment, the meaning of human life (and the meaning of religious belief) will not be found in the neurochemistry of human physiology.

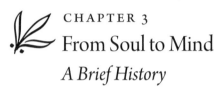

CHAPTER 3

From Soul to Mind

A Brief History

FOR MOST OF human history, we have cherished the idea that there is a separate immaterial part of each of us—a mind or a soul—that must live somewhere within our body. That has gradually changed with the advent of scientific approaches to mind-body relations. We now view the *mind* as a functional property of the brain, not "something located somewhere." The mind is a firmly embodied process within the *brain*, rather like the program that runs within a computer. However, can the same sort of embodiment be presumed for what we traditionally call the *soul*?

This puzzle over relating mind, brain, and soul has ancient roots. Early theories about where to locate the mind varied greatly. Some argued for the heart, some for the brain, and others for the ventricles, the prominent spaces within the brain. We have had a similarly long history with the idea that our soul is a nonmaterial part residing somewhere within us. Generally in history, we have spoken with great confidence about what we think our minds are doing, but that is not the case with the soul. What possible role could it play in conscious life?

The Hebrew and Christian scriptures are an early treasure trove of material about this relationship. But even this rich source does not offer a simple and unified picture. Surprisingly, the scriptures offer not a single mention of the brain, although they contain many references to the soul—and to the spirit, heart, mind, head, face, throat, or stomach, for example. This same conundrum shows up in much of the ancient philosophical literature: where to locate the mind/soul, if anywhere at all?

An early debate arose between some who located the mind/soul in the heart and others who believed it lived inside the brain. In the fifth century BC, the Greek philosopher Empedocles reasserted the notion that the soul (the Greek word for the *mind*) was found in the heart and in the blood, a theory labeled "the cardiovascular theory." But Empedocles' views did not go unchallenged. Around the same time, Alcmaeon of Croton asserted that mental functions are located in the brain. His view was labeled "the encephalic view." For two thousand years, these two theories competed with each other. The great physician, Hippocrates, who lived sometime between 460 and 360 BCE, adopted the brain or encephalic theory of mind. His text *On the Sacred Disease* dealt extensively with epilepsy. He argued that epilepsy is not really a sacred event, but rather an understandable disease with natural causes. Hippocrates also decided that the brain was the interpreter of consciousness and the mediator of feelings.

In the fourth century BCE, the encephalic and cardiovascular theories continued their rivalry in the viewpoints of Plato and Aristotle. Plato seems to have wanted it both ways, locating the immortal soul in the marrow of the head (presumably the brain) but locating the passion between the neck and the midriff. He put the appetites at the navel. For his part, Aristotle quite unambiguously localized the soul in the heart. He had good reasons for his views, which still preserved a role for the brain. Being a good biologist, he noticed that the brain was moist to the touch and concluded that it refrigerated the blood. Aristotle's views were passed on through the Stoic philosophers to one of the early church fathers, Tertullian. The encephalic theory survived through one of Rome's outstanding physicians, Galen.

With Galen, we see the first significant departure from the simpler heart/brain controversy. An accomplished anatomist, Galen provided support for his views with anatomical data from his brain dissections. His detailed examination of the brain impressed him with the size and location of the ventricles, the large spaces within each cerebral hemisphere. He concluded that the so-called "vital spirits" or "animal spirits" of a sentient being must move within this network of ventricles.

Shortly after Galen died, the Germanic invasions in Europe nearly obliterated the Greek and Roman research on the mind, although some of it survived. In the fourth century CE, for example, Bishop Nemesius of Syria claimed to be a loyal follower of Galen, producing a new physical theory of the mind. He defined three different mental faculties—sensation and imagination, thought and judgment, and memory—and then localized each in the different ventricles of the brain. A few centuries later, the ideas of Aristotle and Galen were reintroduced into Europe when they were discovered in manuscripts and translations in Spain. So now there were three groups of partisans, each supporting the encephalic, the cardiovascular, and the ventricular theories of the mind-body relationship.

In the early seventeenth century, Galileo gained fame for his use of empirical evidence to challenge the cosmological beliefs of the Catholic Church. Less well known, his contemporary, Vesalius, was conducting dissections of the human body, including the brain (previously forbidden on theological grounds). He pioneered the empirical approach to the mind-body problem. By dissected the brains of humans, apes, dogs, horses, sheep, and other animals, Vesalius showed that they all possessed ventricles. At the time, Christian anthropology asserted that ventricles were the probable home of the unique human mind and soul, a biological theory that now collapsed. The growing knowledge of anatomy and physiology delivered a similar fate to the cardiovascular theory, discredited finally by William Harvey's analysis of the circulation of the blood.

TRIUMPH OF THE ENCEPHALIC THEORY

Though not without occasional challenges, a general encephalic view became widely accepted. The search now became one of finding out where the mind operated inside the brain. There were just two options: either the mind functioned in specific spots, or it functioned across the entire territory of the brain. This continues to be the great debate in neuroscience. As we shall see, this debate has created one school of thought that has tried to localize brain function, at one time interpreting the brain by bumps on the head (called phrenology), and, more currently, trying to do the same by finding local functions in the brain, including a so-called "God spot" for religious experience.

This attempt at finding a physical spot began famously with the French philosopher René Descartes. He said the soul made contact with the brain in the pineal gland, because, among other things, it was located in the center of the brain. He stated this mostly plainly in his 1649 work, *The Passions of the Soul*, just before he died. Sometime later, in 1664, the distinguished English physiologist Thomas Willis (after whom the "circle of Willis" is named) chose the corpus striatum to locate the soul. Around the same time, French anatomist Raymond Vieussens decided that the centrum semiovale was the right place, and, about fifty years later, the Italian physician Giovanni Lancisi suggested that the mind or the soul should be located in the corpus callosum. As these cases suggest, scientists in the past used whatever tools they had to find local function in the brain. This search has accelerated with the new brain imaging technology. The perennial quest for "localization," however, has also stirred dissent from those who take a more global view of brain functions.

That global outlook was exemplified early on by the French physiologist Jean Pierre Flourens. He did experiments in which he destroyed parts of the cortex of animals. In most cases, there was a pattern of loss and recovery, leading Flourens to conclude that the brain functioned as a whole—mental functions were not localized in particular areas of the cortex. In the early part of the twentieth century, similar experiments were done by Harvard psychologist Karl Lashley, who was trying (but failed) to find the location of the memory for a maze in the cerebral cortex of a rat. Lashley essentially came to the same conclusion as Flourens.

In rebuttal to such a global view, the advocates of localized brain functions have produced their own experimental evidence. Even before Flourens did his work, the Italian physiologist Giovanni Aldini showed that stimulation of the exposed brains of oxen "could produce movements of the eyelids, lips and eyes." In effect, electrical stimulation of different places on the brain would elicit different responses. This research was a follow-up to the work of his uncle, Luigi Galvani, professor of anatomy in Bolonga, who, in 1791, had shown that electricity could excite nerves and muscles. This led him to the claim that "animal electricity," not "animal spirits," was the substance secreted by the brain. There was no longer a need to invoke "immaterial spirits" to move the material body.

Perhaps surprisingly, some scientists and doctors still insisted that the brain had no effect at all on human abilities, such as speech. In 1783, for example, the famous English lexicographer Dr. Samuel Johnson suffered a stroke (detailed in his diaries), and the doctors excluded brain damage from his diagnosis. They instead prescribed a folk treatment that inflicted blisters on each side of his throat, one on his head, and one on his back. They also gave him regular doses of hartshorn, or ammonium carbonate. Thus, the "treatment" showed their belief that the surfaces of the neck and throat were the physical basis of speech. For them, brain events and the mental events involved in speech were not linked. In the years following Johnson's quaint, if painful, experience, the views of medicine would rapidly change, and the debate between global and local brain functions dominated the field.

For the localization camp, a kind of turning point came in the work of Jean Baptiste Bouillard, a contemporary of Flourens. From

his observation of patients with brain damage, Bouillard concluded that "if the brain did not consist of separate centres it would
be impossible to understand how a lesion in one part of the brain
causes paralysis of some muscles of the body without affecting
others."[1] Bouillard believed that localization applied to the understanding of more complex processes like speech.

Following on the work of Bouillard, Marc Dax argued in 1835 that
speech disorders were linked to lesions of the left hemisphere. This
view was further reinforced in 1861, when French neurologist Paul
Broca reported the case of a patient who stopped speaking when
pressure was applied to the left anterior lobes of his brain. Thus, the
notion of cerebral dominance of language in the left hemisphere
was enunciated. German neurologist Karl Wernicke (1874) provided further evidence that even different aspects of language and
speech were localized in different parts of the brain.

During the 1870s, Gustav Fritsch, an anatomist, and Eduard
Hitzig, a psychiatrist, carried out experiments in which they stimulated the cerebral cortex of a dog with electric current to show for
the first time that, by stimulating certain cortical areas, there were
contractions of specific muscles. They claimed that these experiments demonstrated that the cerebral cortex contains "motor
centers." Further research on vision in animals, by lesioning the
visual cortex of a dog, showed that, while the dog could still see, it
could no longer recognize objects. From this time onward, careful
research on animals, together with astute clinical observations by
neurologists, were to build up a picture confirming localization of
function within the brain.

In England, physiologist David Ferrier explored the cerebral
cortex both by stimulation and by judiciously placed lesions. He
showed, for example, that the sense of smell depends on a region
at the tip of the temporal lobe. This substantiated English neurologist John Hughlings-Jackson's observations that hallucinations of
smell often accompanied epileptic fits that arose from tumors in
the same temporal lobe. Nevertheless, Ferrier argued for a medical

distinction between a symptom that arises from a lesion (such as hallucinatory smell) and a local function such as language. He believed that a symptom and a function operated on different cerebral organizations.

Debates between the localists and globalists have continued well into the twentiy-first century. Some neuroscientists today explore examples of tightly constrained local functions in the brain. Others probe the concept of neural networks and parallel distributed processing. They emphasize the unbelievably complex interconnections and interactions between adjacent and distant parts of the brain. In either case, the older belief that mind is separate from the brain has been completely overturned. Today, we recognize the links between brain events and mind events. What is more, data are rapidly accumulating that support a link between brain and personality, including social and ethical behavior.

PHRENOLOGY: MAPPING THE BRAIN

One of the most colorful episodes in this long search for the mind in the brain was the rise of phrenology. It was the first great leap forward in the attempt to localize mental characteristics. After it emerged in the early nineteenth century, phrenology survived for a remarkably long period before it was discredited. It originated in the work of German physicians Franz Joseph Gall and Johann Casper Spurzheim. They identified twenty-seven different mental faculties with areas on the surface of the skull and, therefore, by inference, to underlying brain areas. In this sense, phrenology was both an encephalic and a localizationist model. Persons were thought to have greater or lesser endowment of a particular faculty if there seemed to be a bump or enlargement of that area of the skull.

Between 1820 and 1850, some of the proponents of phrenology, together with those of another fashionable topic, Mesmerism, founded journals to prove and popularize their claims. Their views very soon entered the marketplace. At local fairs and markets, you could have the bumps on your scalp analyzed to discover your special skills and defects. The chief popularizer of phrenology in Britain was the Scottish lawyer George Combe. He learned about phrenology when he attended one of Spurzheim's early lectures in Edinburgh. He was particularly interested in applying phrenology to the reform of society and morals.

Before Franz Gall's empirical work on the brain and head shape, psychology was largely a branch of philosophy and epistemology. No attempt had yet been made to divide the brain into functional regions and to relate these to behavior. Gall pioneered the attempt to use objective measurement to link brain function to behavior. He argued that we should look to external nature rather than personal introspection to classify mental and behavioral phenomena. The goal of his research was "to found a doctrine of the functions of the brain," hoping that "the result of this doctrine ought to be the development of a perfect knowledge of human nature."[2]

The phrenology of Gall and Spurzheim shows that, while empirical evidence is necessary in science, it can also be used to make erroneous claims. To his credit, Gall had collected a massive amount of evidence. His collection of skulls and casts of skulls contained more than six hundred pieces and may still be seen in the Musee de l'Homme in Paris. But a mass of evidence will not guarantee that valid scientific inductions will be made. Gall's naturalism led him into error, and the experimental approach that he rejected would finally win the day. He had adopted a naive inductionist view of science, the so-called Baconian method of gathering facts and then drawing conclusions. In reality, though, Gall had only collected facts that supported his preconceived hypothesis. As historian of science Robert M. Young has written,

> He drew data from each method insofar as it was found to support his initial hypothesis. In short he sought only confirmations. It is not his naturalism that was at fault; it

> is his anecdotal method and the standards of evidence....
> Beginning with Gall, phrenologists have had two charac-
> teristic reactions toward evidence. If it can be construed
> to support phrenology, it is proclaimed as confirmatory.
> If not, it is explained away.[3]

This, in fact, is not an unheard-of procedure (or problem) in research even today.

Gall was not a crank. His views were endorsed by such distinguished investigators as British biologist Alfred Russell Wallace,
codiscoverer of the theory of evolution by natural selection. Apparently, Wallace had read *The Constitution of Man*, a book written
by Combe, the enthusiastic disciple of Gall. The book persuaded
Wallace of the truth of phrenology (he also seems to have believed
the evidence for Mesmerism).

Wallace conducted his own experiments in phrenology and
believed the evidence he obtained was confirmatory. He had his
own head looked at by two phrenologists in 1847 "with such accu-
racy as to render it certain that the positions of all mental organs
had been very precisely determined."[4] Thus convinced, Wallace
needed to explain the contrary findings of David Ferrier on the
effects of local brain lesions. He did this by saying that "the supposed localization of motor areas by Professor Ferrier and others,
which are usually stated to be disproof of the science are really
one of its supports, the movements produced being merely those
which expressed emotions due to the excitation of the phrenological organ excited."[5] As Young comments, "the fact that Wallace
could hold these views further highlights the dangers when the naturalistic method of study is the only one used."[6]

This was also the case with Wallace's own theory of evolution
by natural selection. Wallace, like Darwin, had used a very great
number of naturalistic observations, as well as pieces of anecdotal
evidence, in support of his theory. For most of the nineteenth century, their evolutionary theory was in much the same position as

phrenology, resting as it did on naturalistic observations and the massive set of anecdotes collected more or less systematically. Evidence clinching the evolutionary theory ultimately was available when it was confirmed by the experimental production of varieties by selection. In the case of phrenology, however, no experimental confirmation was forthcoming.

PHRENOLOGY MEETS CHRISTIAN BELIEF

Gall and Spurzheim soon discovered that they had opened themselves to charges of religious infidelity. Gall left Vienna in 1802 when he was accused of advocating materialism and fatalism. This happened despite his assertions about God and his careful description of his methodology. "I leave unsought the nature of the soul as well as the body. . . . I confine myself to phenomena," he wrote of his method. "The object of my research . . . is the brain." One of Gall's favorite mottos was "God and the Brain: Nothing but God and the Brain." Writing in *On Innate Dispositions* (*Des disposition innees*), he explained his scientific ambitions this way: "If we can demonstrate that a relationship exists between the exercise of the soul properties and the origination of their existence in the brain it would no longer be possible to doubt that it is possible to establish a doctrine which will enable us to know the noblest part of the organism."[7]

The historian Robert Rieber has argued that Gall's statement about God and the brain is an example of a pantheistic worldview (in which God is viewed as present in matter).[8] This view clashed with the Catholic Church in Austria, which embraced the Thomistic theory that the soul was above matter and the cause of its life. According to Rieber, Gall seemed to argue that "living bodies are the result of the union of the body and soul."[9] The leaders of the Church in Vienna saw Gall's unified theory of mind-body as a threat to the notion of free will and also to the clergy's responsibility to guide Catholics toward proper moral conduct. Hence, Gall was forced to leave Vienna and flee to Paris. In Rieber's view, "Gall was struggling, either consciously or unconsciously, with how to reconcile a holistic, monistic, theoretical concept of the organism, with an elementalistic mind/brain faculty type of psychology."[10]

If this assessment is correct, then we can see Gall's dilemma as a foreshadowing of current debates about the impact of neuropsychology on some widely held traditional religious views of human nature. Meanwhile, Spurzheim sought to defend himself against similar charges when he wrote *A View of the Philosophical Principles of Phrenology*, in which he invoked Saint Augustine in his defense.[11] However, the pressures on him remained and he moved to Britain to continue his advocacy of phrenology.

The project to Christianize phrenology soon became widespread. Between 1820 and 1860, there were Christian advocates of phrenology on both sides of the Atlantic. When Spurzheim lectured in Edinburgh in 1817, George Combe was in the audience. Two years later, he established the Edinburgh Phrenological Society. By 1838, Combe had written his most famous work, *The Constitution of Man*, which drew heavily upon phrenology. Combe, like many Edinburgh intellectuals, was heavily influenced by the Enlightenment. Phrenology, the so-called new "science of man," afforded another critique of Christianity in the Enlightenment tradition of emphasizing the importance of reason in establishing beliefs.

Around the same time (1833), Orson Fowler graduated from Amherst College in Massachusetts with plans to enter Lane Theological Seminary that fall. During the summer, however, he found that he could earn money lecturing on phrenology and giving character readings of his classmates' heads for two cents each. With $40 in his pocket, he abandoned the idea of ministry and started out on the phrenology circuit. His approach was practical: he used phrenology to give advice on marriage, education, child rearing, and intellectual improvement. For Fowler, British phrenology was too theoretical, "too anxious on a scientific and philosophical basis, to the neglect of practical examinations." In 1843, he published *The Christian Phrenologist*, with the alternative title *The Natural Theology and Moral Bearings of Phrenology: Its Aspect on, and Harmony with Revelation.*

Combe came from a Scottish Calvinist tradition; Fowler was within the American populist Protestant tradition with evangelical overtones. Keeping in mind these differing traditions, it is interesting to explore how these two men sought to relate their shared enthusiasm for phrenology with their religious beliefs.

Combe used his knowledge of phrenology to answer a question that preoccupied him, "How does God govern the world?" Therefore, he probed how the brain (as described by phrenology) produced natural religion and morality—a view influenced by his Enlightenment thinking and, in particular, by deism. "The world is material, man's nature is material, and the whole relation between them depends on the material conditions," he declared. His so-called "spiritual hypothesis" leaned toward materialism, although Combe still believed that God had revealed himself in Scripture as well as through nature. In his study of Combe's belief, psychologist Wayne Norman concludes, "Combe came to phrenology as a deist and argued for deism from phrenological principles. . . . Thus, Combe's critique of Christianity can be seen as an argument for the replacement of orthodox Christian doctrine with deistic principles."[12]

Norman argues that Fowler was also seeking a scientific basis for religion. There is no indication that Fowler ever rejected Christianity, he says, but Fowler was nevertheless deeply concerned to counter sectarianism. Although Fowler questioned a number of orthodox doctrines and elevated reason over revelation, according to Norman, he also sought to purify Christianity. Norman notes that many phrenologists tried to reconcile their science with a Christian faith. In 1835, for example, the Christian minister Henry Clarke of Dundee, Scotland, published *Christian Phrenology*; or

The Teachings of the New Testament Respecting the Animal, Moral and Intellectual Nature of Man. He saw phrenology as a friend to Christianity.

In a similar vein, the British physician Charles Cowan in 1841 published his *Phrenology Consistent with Science and Revelation.* He championed a harmony between divinely revealed scripture and the science of phrenology. Since the same God rules nature and revelation, he argued, science and religion must ultimately be in harmony. Belief in the immortality of the soul, he added, is based on revelation, not science. Similarly, phrenology cannot interfere with revealed truths. Yet another phrenology reconciler was W. Easton, who wrote a book entitled *The Harmony of Phrenology with Scripture on the Doctrine of the Soul.* Easton believed that "the truths of Nature discovered by science must be respected, and Scripture must accommodate itself to these truths."[13]

Theologically, the most conservative of the Christian phrenologists was William Scott. He held a high view of Christian revelation, yet at the same time wanted to vindicate phrenology. The title of his book, *The Harmony of Phrenology with Scripture,* reflects his beliefs—some of which sound very modern. For example, the soul (or self) is a "simple and indivisible being of which the brain is the organ during life." Of the phrenological faculties, he wrote that they are "merely different states of this simple being; that the separate organs of the brain afford the means by which these states of mind are induced and manifested."[14]

By considering the views of this small sample of nineteenth-century Christians who sought to relate the "brain science" of phrenology with their Christian beliefs, we find a wide variety of proffered solutions. Some wanted to "replace" religion with science (Combe), some to "purify" religion (Fowler), some to find in science a "friend and helpmate" (Clarke), and some to "harmonize" science and faith (Cowan and Scott). All of these positions are echoed in modern writings about the relationships between psychology, neuroscience, and religious belief.

FINDING THE "GOD SPOT":
THE NEW PHRENOLOGY?

Today's dramatic new results in brain research, known to us in eye-catching multicolored pictures from brain scans, are reminiscent of the old phrenology maps showing "spiritual bumps" on the head. Using the latest brain-imaging techniques, the "new phrenologists" are on the same quest to identify the part or parts of our brains most active when we are meditating, praying, or seeking contact with the transcendent. The earliest contemporary studies focused on how epileptic seizures in the temporal lobe seemed linked, in some patients, to experiencing religious awe, a cosmic presence, or visions. Of course, this was eventually popularized as a discovery of the "God spot" in the brain.

One of the earliest volumes relating brain structures to the search for the sacred was the provocatively titled *Where God Lives in the Human Brain* (2001). The authors, Carol Albright and James Ashbrook, believed that they had begun to identify the elusive "God spot" and suggested that it is possible that we are indeed hardwired to seek God. For example, they wrote, "All that may be new here is an analysis that finds in the human brain a mirror of these *imagines dei*—all these images of God—and thus may suggest further ways of comprehending them."[15] Christian phrenologist Henry Clarke would have approved of this.

A more recent advocate of the temporal lobe as the elusive "God spot" is writer and researcher Willoughby Britton. Reporting on Britton's work, Julia Keller wrote, "The temporal lobe, Britton said, is considered 'the God module,' the part of the brain that connects with the transcendent."[16] Others look elsewhere in the brain. Osamu Muramoto, a research neurologist, describes his interest in the causes of people being hyper religious. He writes, "Hyperreligiosity may stem from increased activity in the medial prefrontal cortex of the brain. . . . My theory is that the medial prefrontal cortex plays the role of the conductor of an orchestra in religiosity."[17]

All of this neurological study of religious experience has resulted in people talking about a new field of research called *neurotheology*. Indeed, some researchers have even tried to draw conclusions about the truth of religious claims from the study of biological brain events. Others are far more cautious in presuming interpretations. For example, Mario Beauregard, who works in the departments of Radiology and Psychology at the Université de Montreal, offers this: "Obviously, the external reality of God can neither be confirmed nor disconfirmed by delineating neural correlates of religious/spiritual/mystical experiences. In other words, the neuroscientific study of what happens to the brain during these experiences does not tell us anything new about God."[18] Christian phenologist William Scott would have applauded this sentiment.

The distinguished Jewish physician Jerome Groopman expressed his concerns about some of the motivations for neurotheology when he wrote, "Why do we have this strange attempt, clothed in the rubric 'neurotheology,' to objectify faith with the bells and whistles of technology?" He went on, "Man is a proper subject for study in the world of science. God is not." Groopman acknowledges that, while the idea of humans being intrinsically wired for spirituality cannot be summarily dismissed, he cautions that, "as has been the case with all attempts to 'prove' the presence or intent of God, [brain] scans and cerebral anatomy fall far short of doing so." And he concludes, "Indeed to believe that science is a way to decipher the divine, that technology can capture God's photograph, is to deify man's handiwork. And that, both religious mystics and scholars agree, is the essence of idolatry."[19]

We saw earlier how Combe sought to use phrenology to influence other domains of knowledge and behavior (in his case, the reform of society and morals). Today, some people seem to be using neurotheology to prove theological truths. Similarly, Fowler attempted to find a scientific basis for religion from phrenology. We have apparently not learned the lesson that it is unwise to try to bolster faith with current science. For those who relied on phrenology to have faith, what happened when phrenology turned out to be wrong? Phrenology seemed to provide "scientific evidence" for "spiritual bumps" on the brain's surface, proving the reality of the spiritual. If our modern society had remembered the story of phrenology, we might have been spared the current enthusiasm to, as Groopman says, "objectify faith with the bells and whistles of technology."

LESSONS FROM HISTORY

The long search to locate the soul/mind "somewhere" in the body is rich with lessons. Many of those lessons are simply being revived by modern attempts to find the brain location of each human experience, especially in the trend we have called *neurotheology*. The work of Joseph Gall, the pioneer phrenologist, offers us four lessons on why today's neurotheology faces pitfalls in its technological attempts to find a biological basis of religious experience.

The first lesson is this: although Gall's work showed great skill at collecting empirical evidence about the human skulls, he failed to undertake experiments to test his conclusions. He used an admirable naturalistic approach but never investigated his hypothesis. The failure to do this adequately was the Achilles heel of Gall's formidable research. Second, Gall's work was always in danger of slipping into an unthinking reductionism, as is some neurotheology. To his credit, however, Gall did try to understand our complex mental functions before attempting to link them to the brain. He foreshadowed the excellent work of Donald Hebb, one of the twentieth century's most distinguished psychologists.

The third lesson we draw from Gall's work is salutary. He was very wise to conclude that the physical findings of brain science are extremely limited when trying to draw theological conclusions. As he wrote,

> The investigator of nature can only fathom the laws of the world of the body and takes for granted that no natural truth could be inconsistent with any revealed one.

Beyond this, he knows that . . . he has nothing to decide about mental life. He only sees and teaches that in this life mind is bound to body organisation.[20]

Robert Rieber has analyzed Gall's writings and presents us with a fourth lesson from phrenology—a lesson relevant to the ambitions of neurotheology. Hidden in Gall's work was an assumption about material constraints on free will, a view that conflicted with long-held dogmas of the Catholic Church. Rieber believes that Gall's unified theory of mind and body was indeed a threat to the classic notion of free will, to which we shall return later in the book.

Overall, we can see that the era of phrenology produced a variety of reactions among Christian leaders, all of them drawing different conclusions for religious beliefs and practice. George Combe, for example, used phrenology as an Enlightenment critique of Christianity and as a support for his deist beliefs. In contrast, Orson Fowler saw phrenology as a helpful tool for practical pastoral matters such as marriage, education, and child rearing. Charles Cowan believed that scripture must accommodate itself to the truths of nature. William Scott, much like Gall, believed that there was a harmony between phrenology and scripture. With phrenology, as with the information being revealed by modern neuroscience, there is a wide variety of possible relationships between science and one's religious faith.

As this survey reveals, the empirical and reductionist approach of phrenology is not as old-fashioned as it seems. The general public is regaled almost daily with dramatic pictures from brain imaging that claim to show separate parts of the brain selectively active for almost every conceivable human activity. Science has indeed begun to show us discreet modules in the brain for each possible mental capacity. Nevertheless, the story is always more complicated, and that leads us to looking at the more complex models of the brain offered to us today by the best science.

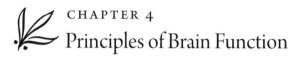

CHAPTER 4
Principles of Brain Function

ALTHOUGH THE BRAIN can be thought of in terms of parts, modules, and systems, it also may be understood by its varied principles of operation. These principles can guide our understanding of broader psychological issues. By understanding these principles—and we shall outline eight that we feel are most helpful—we can begin to talk about how neuroscience is finding ever-tighter links between the functioning of our brain systems and our mental lives.

1. ACTION LOOPS

The nervous system is, in its simplest form, an action loop. The basic task for the nervous systems of all organisms is to adjust its ongoing motor activity based on sensory consequences. The nervous system modulates actions in the world by using sensory systems to monitor action outcomes, comparing actual outcomes to intended outcomes, and, on the basis of this feedback, making adjustments to ongoing action. This process results in the constant cycling of an action–feedback–evaluation–action loop (see Figure 1).

This principle reveals that it is the nature of organisms to be involved in constant interaction with their surroundings, always moving toward biologically relevant goals. Thus, even in the case of human beings, it is not so much that we stop-and-calculate and then act, but rather we are constantly acting (in some form) and making adjustments to actions based on feedback. Consequently, the basic problem for the brain is efficient and effective action-in the world. Our subjective thought and cognition are derived from this action processing, including all the complex levels involved in modulating ongoing action.

2. A Nested Hierarchy of Action Loops

As we move upward from the brain stem to the cerebral cortex, there are new and more complex structures of action-feedback interactions (which we call *sensory-motor*). These structures create a hierarchy of action loops—that is, lower-level loops are nested within, and modulated by, higher-level loops. The nested hierarchy involves (or is constituted by) various forms of feed-forward and feedback between levels. By *levels*, we mean (at least as a rough outline for immediate discussions) the anatomical division of the nervous system into spinal cord, brain stem, midbrain, diencephalon (that is, structures and nuclei lying just beneath the cerebral cortex), and the cerebral cortex.

Figure 2 gives a simple diagram of what we have in mind. Each higher level (box) involves more complex forms of modulation of lower levels. Thus, as a simplified model, action loops within the spinal cord are controlled and modulated by being nested within higher-level loops involving areas of the brain stem, while brain stem systems are nested within control loops involving midbrain systems. So, an important basic principle of brain function is to imagine increasingly higher and more complex nesting of the control of action—that is, a nested control hierarchy.

The idea of levels of nesting is not limited to the very gross divisions of the nervous system represented in Figure 2. The cerebral cortex (the highest-level box in this diagram) also embodies a nested hierarchy of sensory-motor interactions. You can see this hierarchy in the diagram of Figure 3. The cerebral cortex has "lower-level" areas performing more immediate sensory processing (the primary processing areas for vision, audition, touch, etc.) and "lower-level" areas for the immediate motor output. These areas interact with areas doing higher (or more complex) forms of specific sensory processing (often called *sensory association areas*) and areas providing higher levels of motor processing (called the *premotor* and *supplementary motor cortices*). These secondary levels interact, in turn, with the most complex levels of polymodal sensory processing (found in posterior cortex—the inferior temporal cortex and posterior parietal lobe). The motor areas of the cortex are under hierarchical modulatory control from the prefrontal cortex that does the most complex forms of analysis of outcomes versus intentions and long-term behavioral planning.

It is important to point out that, while the cerebral cortex of a human is somewhat larger than that of a chimpanzee, the most remarkable difference is the relatively large size of the posterior polymodal association cortex and the prefrontal cortex in humans. Thus, one part of the story of human cognitive power is greater size and complexity at the top of the hierarchy of action loops.

3. Off-line Action Emulation

If we reflect on our own thinking process, it may be hard to believe that it is a "modulation of sensory-motor loops," as outlined in Figure 3. However, current research suggests that our highest levels of thought do indeed piggy-back on these cortical-sensory and motor-control systems by running them off-line (that is, without consequences for current behavior). Thus, the highest levels of human cognition can be thought of (somewhat simplistically, but nevertheless helpfully) as running the highest levels of action loops in off-line simulations of physical events, such as sight, sound, or speech. We can trigger activity in our cortical sensory systems to elicit images and sensory memories by our prefrontal cortex activating off-line parts of our cortical-sensory apparatus, or we can simulate potential actions, including speech acts, by off-line interactions between the frontal cortex and our cortical-motor systems.

All of this allows human beings to think, imagine, and problem-solve "in the head" by internally simulating relevant actions (including inner speech acts).

4. ESSENTIAL SUPPORT SYSTEMS

Figures 2 and 3 represent one possible model of how the brain functions to accomplish effective and efficient behavior. However, there are brain structures and systems that are not well represented within this form of diagrammatic model. The most interesting of these structures immediately underlie the cerebral cortex. It is helpful to have in mind the names and general properties of these structures.

The basal ganglia are a series of structures that serve to regulate motor behavior. They function to initiate new behaviors, inhibit behaviors, and coordinate action by modulating their speed and amplitude. An example of the role played by these structures is seen in disorders like Huntington's disease and Parkinson's disease. The basal ganglia is not the only structure that controls motor behavior: there is also the cerebellum, down in the area of the midbrain. The cerebellum, however, seems to be more dedicated to the timing and coordination of rapid motor actions in particular.

Another important brain area is the hippocampus, lying just below the medial surface of the temporal lobe. This structure is critical for the formation of new memories of life events. Information from much of the cerebral cortex flows into the hippocampus (and the immediately adjacent cortical areas) and then back out to the cortex to cause consolidation of the cortical networks that represent (or "remember") the experience, thus enabling access to the memory at some later time. Persons with damage to the hippocampus (on both sides of the brain) have amnesia, that is, severe problems with forming new memories.

The amygdala lies within the anterior temporal lobe and is an important area for emotions, particularly fear. In a sense, the amygdala is an important station on a parallel path to the cortex, getting input from lower brain systems and providing the cortex and other structures with information with respect to the biological or personal significance of potentially fear-relevant environmental stimuli.

Finally, there is a part of the cerebral cortex that is considered very ancient in the evolution of the human brain: it is often referred to as limbic cortex (suggesting its important role in emotions and evaluation of the significance of information). This cortex forms a continuous inner ring but has different names at different parts of the ring. One area is called medial temporal cortex, while another is called cingulate cortex (divided into anterior and posterior portions). Limbic cortex is phylogenetically older and less complex (fewer cellular layers) than the rest of the cerebral cortex.

In summary, the control hierarchy diagrammed for the entire brain (Figure 2) and, more specifically, within a hierarchical model of the cerebral cortex (Figure 3) is supplemented by processes occurring in other structures and systems: basal ganglia and cerebellum (motor), hippocampus (memory), amygdala (fear), and limbic cortex (emotional significance).

5. Localization of Function within the Brain

The concept of "localization of function" generally refers to the fact that the brain is not one large undifferentiated processing mass. Rather, it is organized into areas responsible for certain functions. Such localization is very distinct in structures of the brain below the level of the cerebral cortex—both with respect to the clearly identified functions of areas within the brain stem, midbrain, and thalamus, and to the supplementary, subcortical areas described above. In most all of these lower brain areas, distinctly bounded regions can be clearly seen. These are the modules of "gray matter," made up of nerve cells called *nuclei*. The pathways and tracts that interconnect the gray matter areas are also quite visible as "white matter." In the vast majority of cases, a fairly distinct form of functional processing can be identified for these regions. So, for example, there are the cochlear nuclei of the brainstem that do very primitive forms of processing of auditory information; or the superior colliculi in the midbrain that take in visual information and do spatial calculations that allow for eye-tracking and head orientation; or the subcortical nucleus of the amygdala described above.

Localization of function in the lower brain is uncontroversial. The controversy arises over finding the location of various high-level human cognitive capacities in the cerebral cortex. This theoretical pendulum has swung back and forth over the last two centuries, going from a very modular/localizationist view of cortical processing at one pole to a very holistic view at the other pole. While the primary sensory and motor areas (the lower boxes on Figure 3) are clearly localized and have functions that are easy to describe, researchers have acute disagreements about brain functions outside these primary cortical areas.

Two further points are helpful to keep in mind with respect to localization of function within the cerebral cortex. First, modern research using functional magnetic resonance imagining (fMRI) is consistently producing results showing a small number of specific cortical areas that are involved in rather specific and high-level human mental states and experiences, such as contemplating moral dilemmas or observing faces or formulating speech. For example, the localization of processing within the cerebral cortex is evident in the fMRI images of Figure 4 from the research of Michael Spezio and colleagues.[1] Superimposed on the lateral surfaces of the right and left hemisphere are red patches that designate areas of the brain that are reliably (over an entire group of persons) more active during focused attention (or mindfulness) when compared to situations in which the persons' minds are wandering and they are not paying attention. In the top pair of images, the person is asked to concentrate on a voice being heard over earphones in a dry reading of a narrative (actually, reading from Charles Darwin's *Voyage of the Beagle*). When the person is concentrating and mindful of the passage being read, activity in the cerebral cortex is increased (indicated in red) in parietal and frontal areas (mostly on the left side of the brain). Most interesting are the bottom images. Here the same persons (who happened to be long-time practitioners of Christian centering prayer) are engaging in their meditative practice. When they are focused on their meditation, cortical activity is again enhanced in parietal and frontal areas, but now only on the right side and more extensive in the frontal lobes. The right hemisphere is thought to be more involved in processing emotions and information related to the self. For our purposes at this juncture, the main point is that various forms of human mental activity are associated with patterns of localized enhanced neural activity.

So, fMRI research seems to support the localizationist view. However, detractors would want to point out that the fMRI images that appear to reveal focal areas of activity are always representations of the areas that are more active during a particular mental state of interest to investigators compared to some other state not of interest. This process of highlighting only relatively more active regions blurs the fact that most of the cortex is active to some degree during most mental states.

This relates to the second point about localization of function. Many neuroscientists believe that what appear to be modules of localized processing are actually serving as important nodes, or connection points, in an otherwise widely distributed processing network. Thus, the processing related to any particular higher cognitive capacity is not entirely localized in a particular module but unevenly spread over the entire cortex, with certain nodes in the network more highly active and more important to the processing than others. The idea of critical nodes in wider networks represents an intermediate position between the strong localizationist and holist views.

In either case, however, the more that high-level human cognition is found "localized" in particular cortical regions (whether as processing modules or nodes in wider networks), the stronger becomes the argument for a link between brain function and human mind.

6. GENETIC BLUEPRINTS VERSUS A SELF-ORGANIZING BRAIN

Another principle that is important regarding the human brain is the difference between fixed brain structures and functions (that is, as if determined by a genetic blueprint) and the more plastic and self-organizing functional aspects of cortical processing. The large-scale anatomy of the brain is the same in every normal individual. With respect to overall shape, as well as the location and size of the distinct regions and pathways, the brain of one person looks pretty much like the brain of another. In addition, the lower-brain and subcortical regions function in much the same way in all normal individuals. Thus, these structural and functional aspects of the brain are genetically determined.

While the wrinkled surface of the cerebral cortex varies somewhat from person to person, the location of major cortical areas is also largely invariant between persons. Thus, such structures as the visual cortex, motor cortex, and language processing areas are in the same locations in almost all persons, presuming no abnormal prenatal and postnatal events. This suggests that even the rough functional organization of the cerebral cortex is strongly influenced (or predisposed) by genetics.

However, despite this rough functional organization, humans are born with a cerebral cortex that is markedly immature in terms of the number of neurons, complexity of neuron branches, connections between neurons (synapses), and the development of long-distant axon pathways. The human cerebral cortex takes significantly longer to complete its physical development than the

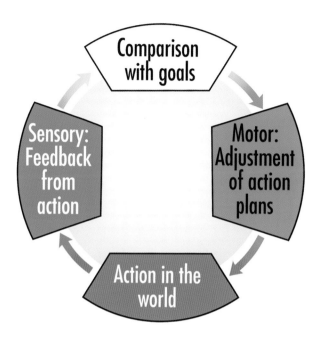

FIGURE 1. The action loop

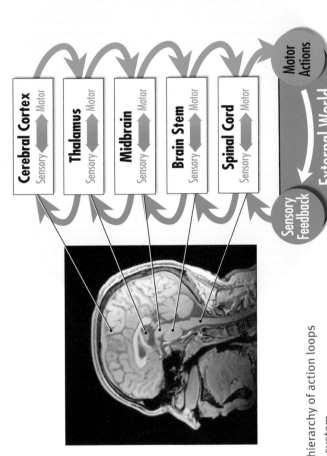

Figure 2. The nested hierarchy of action loops of the human nervous system

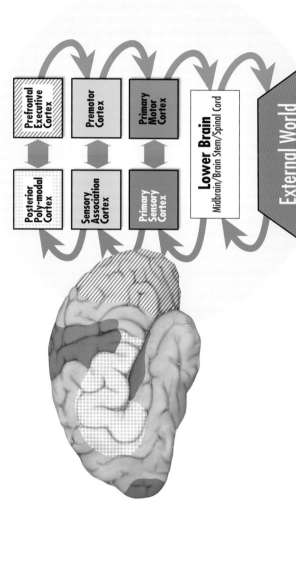

FIGURE 3. The nested hierarchy of action loops of the human cerebral cortex

LEFT HEMISPHERE   RIGHT HEMISPHERE

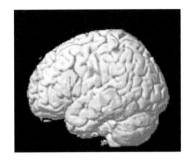 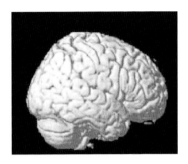

ATTENDING TO NARRATIVE

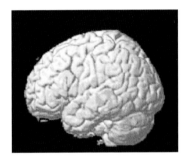 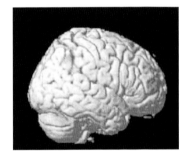

CENTERING PRAYER

FIGURE 4. fMRI images showing areas of enhanced cortical activity (red) while attending to the reading of an academic book (top two images) and while engaging in contemplative prayer (bottom two images)

cortex of young chimpanzees or other primates. The prefrontal cortex, for example, does not reach full adult maturity with respect to cortical thickness or axon myelinization until late in the second decade of life. (Myelinization refers to a process by which axons— somewhat like connecting strands of electrical wire—receive a cellular coating allowing for more rapid and efficient information transmission.)

During the first two to three years of human life, there is a proliferation of nerve branching (dendrites) and connections (synapses), followed by a period of pruning of branches and connections. It is generally believed that the branches and connections that remain are the ones that get incorporated into the networks created by the child's experiences and learning. Thus, the cerebral cortex of a human infant is to some degree functionally self-organizing. As the structures are physically maturing, they are being functionally formed by experiences in the world.

A noteworthy difference between human and chimpanzee infants and children is the very slow maturation of the human cerebral cortex. Thus, the young human brain is distinct for having a long period in which its final neural organization can be influenced by cognitive, social, and cultural experiences.

7. The Brain and Learning

Change does not end with childhood and adolescence, however. Even after the cerebral cortex has reached adult levels of complexity, the functional networks of the cortex remain plastic. They can be modified by new experiences and by learning. This comes about by increased efficiency in initiating and sustaining activity within neural networks. This, in turn, is due to changes in the efficiency of certain synapses (and not others) or formation of new synapses or the growth of new neuronal branches. Thus, the cerebral cortex continues the process of organization and reorganization of functional networks through experiences, learning, imagination, and thought. As already described above, the hippocampus is particularly critical in establishing and modifying the neural networks that constitute learning and memory. Interestingly, the hippocampus is one of the few areas of the brain that continues to receive and incorporate new neurons throughout one's lifetime.

Changes in synaptic efficiency are not limited to the cerebral cortex. Much (but definitely not all) of the brain is susceptible to modification of its functioning due to learning.

8. The Brain and Consciousness

The term *consciousness* has at least two separate meanings when it comes to brain processes. First, there is the idea of being conscious versus being unconscious. This basic form of consciousness is based on interactions between structures of the lower brain (brainstem and midbrain) and the upper brain (particularly the cerebral cortex). Damage to areas of the lower brain can render a person unconscious and functionally vegetative.

The other form of consciousness is the subjective experience of having a stream of mental life that we are aware of—that is, we are conscious of a memory, the person with whom we are talking, a scene we are imagining, etc. No one really knows for sure what creates the specific content of our consciousness, although most would agree that it is a product of the functioning of the cerebral cortex (although strongly influenced by things happening in subcortical structures).

Since our conscious thought is most critical to comprehending the relationship among neuroscience, psychology, and religion, it is important to provide a deeper understanding of this process. Much goes on below the level of conscious awareness in human mental activity, but that which is most critical, and (seemingly) most distinctive of human kind, is what occurs in consciousness.

In our view, the most helpful model of consciousness that modern research has produced is called the "dynamic core hypothesis."

It is well supported by the experimental literature, and it clarifies the difference between the conscious control of behavior and behaviors that are more unconscious and automatic. This model has been ably presented by neuroscientists Gerald Edelman and Giulio Tononi in their book *A Universe of Consciousness: How Matter Becomes Imagination* (2000).

In describing consciousness, Edelman and Tononi suggest a two-part model. Primary (or basic-level) consciousness is evident in the ability of many animals to "construct a mental scene," but this form of consciousness has limited semantic or symbolic content. Higher-order consciousness is "accompanied by a sense of self and the ability, in the waking state, to construct explicit past and future scenes. It requires, at minimum, a semantic capacity and, in its most developed form, a linguistic capacity."[2]

What is most noteworthy about the dynamic core hypothesis is its specification of the most likely neurophysiological basis of conscious awareness. Edelman and Tononi argue that a state of consciousness and its content (whether primary or higher-order) is a temporary and dynamically changing process within the cerebral cortex that is characterized by a high degree of functional interconnectedness among widespread areas. This functional interconnectedness is created by rapid, two-way neural interactions. This widespread functional integration is the "dynamic core," a complex and highly differentiated neural state that changes from moment to moment, including different subsets of neurons at different moments. The specific neural groupings involved, and the functional relations among the groupings, define the nature and content of consciousness at any particular moment. Thus, a particular dynamic core is a functionally interactive subset of the neurons of the cortex; not all of the cerebral cortex is admitted into a dynamic core at any moment.

According to Edelman and Tononi, dynamic cores (and thus consciousness) are characteristic of the mental life of all animals to the degree that the cerebral cortex has sufficiently rich recurrent interconnections. The higher-order consciousness that is distinctive in human beings comes into play when symbolic representations and language are incorporated into dynamic cores, including the ability to represent the self as an abstract entity and to use symbols to note time (past, present, and future). Since language and other symbolic systems are learned, higher-order consciousness is a developmental achievement dependent on social interactions and social scaffolding.

In the early learning of difficult tasks or behaviors, the performance must be incorporated in and regulated by the dynamic core (that is, by consciousness). However, once the behavior is well learned (and automatic), it can go forward efficiently based on the activity of a smaller subgroup of cortical neurons (and subcortical connections) that do not have to be incorporated into the current dynamic core. For example, during normal adult speech, the basic lexical and syntactic aspects of language processing can go on in the background, while the dynamic core embodies the ideas that one is attempting to express.

Our review of the eight principles of brain functioning, ending in the dynamic core model, provides a glimpse of the embodiment of mind. Our highest-level cognition is provided by our cerebral cortex, which forms the top of the control hierarchy of action loops. But it is not just having a cerebral cortex that forms our humanness, but the organization of the cerebral cortex. The highest level of the control hierarchy (in the polymodal cortex and prefrontal cortex) is not only relatively larger in humankind but slower to develop, allowing maximal opportunity for the richness of human society and culture to influence the networks of functional connections.

We believe it is no longer helpful or reasonable to consider mind a nonmaterial entity that can be decoupled from the body. The mind is an active process by which we constantly modulate our action in the world (including the world of human society and culture). Out of continual experiences of action and feedback, the mind becomes formed as a functional property of our brain and body. However, for any of us to accept that our "I" is not a separate inner agent—like the captain of a ship—is a very hard task, counterintuitive to all we know. Next, we will show why this happens.

CHAPTER 5
Linking Mind and Brain

WE ALL HAVE this strong intuition: "I" am an immaterial "thing." We each experience "self" or "mind" separate from the body but inhabiting the body. My intuition is confirmed every day by my friends who share my views—they presume that I have hidden within me a "mind" with intentions, thoughts, and ideas not readily apparent in my behavior. It has also been confirmed by millions of people who have lived down through the ages, some of them the greatest thinkers the world has known.

We could multiply the examples, so strong is this intuition of ourselves. If "I" drink too much alcohol, I lose my grip on "myself." When "I" make decisions in my life, I am in control—control of my thoughts, my actions, my destiny. For that to be possible, I assume that my body, or at least those parts of my body that are most relevant, are reliable. My body is as responsive to "me" as I make use of that machinery every day. I switch on the ignition of my car, and I can be certain, all things being equal, that the engine will spring to life, the wheels turn, and the brakes work. I want this same control over my bodily machinery, and so it is very hard to believe that "I" am my body—that the operation of my body is me.

These kinds of human intuitions can be so strong that even science cannot entirely eliminate them. For example, it once was obvious that the world is flat. Just looking at it, how could I possibly believe that it is round? This is called "phenomenological" evidence—what we actually see and experience—and it is often overwhelming. Our senses say, "My desk is solid." But another kind of knowledge tells us that not only is the world round but my desk is mostly just space—the spaces between the minute particles of which it is made up.

Thus, my intuitions and those I share with millions of others can be wrong. Could it also be that my intuitions about my nature, about my personal make-up, need reexamining? We often know this from direct personal experience. When a close friend suffers a stroke, for example, he no longer seems in full control of his thoughts and actions. But if the real "I" is an immaterial "something" separate from my body, how could this be? Surely anything happening to the body should not touch the immaterial mind or soul?

The scientific enterprise, with its untold benefits for our health and quality of life, has also changed our view of who we are, often at the cost of our strongest intuitions. We have already reviewed this history, from locating the soul/mind in the physical brain, in the debate over local or global processes, and then principles by which the parts of the brain and body seem to cooperate to create consciousness. But contemporary neuroscience is taking us further still. As we review developments in the past half century of brain science, we can see that a whole new series of questions has been posed. In addition to questions about the "fixity" of brain events, we are now asking how much "plasticity"—or potential for change—underlies brain mechanisms. In addition, we want to know whether we can simply "reduce" all of our talk about the mind to descriptions of what is happening in the brain.

The Birth of Neuropsychology

By the eve of World War II, neuroscience harbored no doubts about the strong relationship between mind and brain. The accumulation of evidence for a century or more showed one thing: however you look at it, the brain is the organ of mind.

During the second half of the last century, prompted especially by the aftermath of war, there was a reawakening of interest in the relationship between the brain and behavior. Facing the task of rehabilitating thousands of wounded servicemen, research advanced rapidly. As sometimes happens in science, the outcome was not so much the discovery of new ideas but the rediscovery of old ones. When the views of early twentieth-century neurologists were combined with new behavioral techniques being developed in experimental psychology, a new field of neuropsychology was born—although the term *neuropsychology* seems to have been first used by Sir William Osler in a 1913 address to open the Phipps Clinic at the Johns Hopkins Hospital.

In more recent years, the rapid development of the related field of cognitive neuroscience is generally attributed to the convergence of three separate scientific endeavors: cognitive psychology, comparative neuropsychology, and brain imaging. The cognitive revolution within experimental psychology freed it from its narrow behaviorist approaches, giving rise to the subdiscipline of cognitive psychology—the understanding of mind through scientific observations of behavior. Now, psychologists could talk freely about mental events and not simply about stimulus-response contingencies. The development of new experimental techniques enabled cognitive psychologists to sort mental processes into their component parts—memory, for example, into short-term memory, long-term memory, and working memory.

In comparative neuropsychology, techniques found useful in studying human cognition (remembering and perceiving) were adapted and applied to the study of animals. Exciting early findings came from studies of memory and visual perception. American neurophysiologists David Hubel and Thorsten Wiesel used single-cell recording techniques to study the neural underpinnings of vision in cats, prompting others to follow with similar studies in awake and alert monkeys.[1] The fortuitous discovery by British neuropsychologist Brenda Milner (working in Canada) of the loss of the ability to form new memories due to surgical removal of the hippocampus spawned a whole new scientific industry of studies of the effects of hippocampal damage in animals.[2]

To follow, the noninvasive techniques of magnetic resonance imaging (MRI), positron emission tomography (PET), and functional magnetic resonance imaging (fMRI) were applied to awake humans. While MRIs provide pictures of the anatomical structure of a person's brain, PET and fMRI make it possible to monitor regions of the brain that are more or less active while a person is engaged in specific mental tasks. The newest technique is transcranial magnetic stimulation (TMS), which can temporarily disable regions of the cortex without damage to brain structure. In that sense, its effect is "reversible." The TMS magnetic coil is placed on the outside of the skull so that its magnetic field can simply target (turn off) different cortical areas.

Not surprisingly, progress in neuroscience over the last century was accompanied by swings in its philosophical underpinnings. In the mid-twentieth century, research on brain-damaged humans was combined with studies involving brain lesions in animals, and generally interpreted in the behaviorist framework dominating North American psychology. This gave rise to what neuroscientist and Nobel laureate Roger Sperry described as "the materialist 'micro-determinist' view of nature" in which "all mental and brain functions are determined by, and can be explained by, brain physiology and neuronal activity."[3] This bottom-up approach located all of the causes of behavior at the microlevel of brain function. However, more recent evidence has made this view increasing problematic. As we shall see, research has increasingly supported the possibility of a major top-down causal role for cognitive processes.

Thus, by the 1970s, Roger Sperry argued that there had been a shift in the scientific status and treatment of conscious experience, a shift that would have far-ranging philosophic and humanistic, as well as scientific, implications. He argued that these "mentalistic revisions" in the understanding of human nature "invoke emergent forms of causal control that transform conventional scientific descriptions of both human and nonhuman nature."[4] By believing that the causal role of cognitive processes cannot be "reduced to" isolated brain activity, researchers were not at all restricted in their localization studies of memory, speech, and mental planning, for example. But they also expanded on their holistic interpretation of the brain's higher-mental causes. They viewed them as "emerging" from an ensemble of brain networks, not just a single node or module.

TIGHTENING THE LINKS
OF MIND AND BRAIN

As a result of these recent developments, the research disciplines of cognitive psychology, comparative neuropsychology, and brain imaging generally agree that specific mental processes correlate to regions or systems in the brain. The linkages are particularly well illustrated by three areas of research: the interaction of the left and right halves of the brain, the brain's role in the recognition of human faces, and the way brain injury can influence moral behavior and human personality.

Two Brain Hemispheres
One of the most intensively studied issues has been differences in the structure, and in information processing, between the left and right cerebral hemispheres. It was Sperry's work using the so-called "split-brain preparation" that gave fresh impetus to research on the distinctive roles of the two cerebral hemispheres. As a result of this research, there were rapid advances in understanding how cognitive functions were localized differently in the two cerebral hemispheres.

The split-brain preparation earned its name from experiments on animals in which Ronald Myers and Roger Sperry surgically disconnected the main pathways connecting the brain's two cerebral hemispheres. The same surgical procedure was subsequently applied to a small group of epilepsy patients in whom, as a last resort, the corpus callosum, the major pathway joining the two cerebral hemispheres (and in some cases other smaller connecting pathways), was surgically cut in order to reduce the spread of epileptic signals from one cerebral hemisphere into the other.

In the eighteenth century, authors such as Lancisi believed that the corpus callosum—the "callous body" or "hard part" of the brain—was the seat of the soul. Eventually, research suggested that it might have no function at all. In 1941, neurophysiologists Warren McCulloch and Hugh Garol reported that lesions or surgery of the corpus callosum have "failed to produce any characteristic disorders except, possibly, impairment of coordination of the hemispheres in complicated symbolic activity."[5]

However, careful study by Sperry and his colleagues showed that cutting the corpus callosum in these "split-brain" patients produced major changes in some of their mental activities. Direct awareness was no longer unified. An object placed in the left hand out of sight could not be matched to the same object felt separately and unseen in the right hand. As long as the eyes remained stationary, something seen to the left of a point in space could not be accurately compared to something seen to the right of that point. Similar divisions in olfactory and auditory awareness were also demonstrated. Subsequently, more detailed testing showed that some very general stimulus can transfer between the surgically separated right and left hemispheres, following subcortical pathways. But the basic split-brain findings are well established.

One very dramatic finding of early split-brain research was that the right cerebral cortex of patients could not express itself in speech. The right cortex could know things but not produce words to explain them. By contrast, when stimuli were given to the left cortex, the patient could explain perfectly well what the stimulus had been like. In other words, when the corpus callosum is cut, each hemisphere shows (under appropriate test conditions) a separate world of awareness. There were two minds in one brain.[6]

Today, neuropsychologists recognize that simplistic talk about the hemispheric lateralization of function begs important questions: What is it that is lateralized? Are the cerebral hemispheres differently organized? Do they have two distinct ways of processing information? Despite these remaining puzzles, the study of split-brain patients has revealed much about the different capacities of the two cerebral hemispheres and about the splitting of consciousness. This has also had a remarkable impact on how we understand the relationships between brain processes and mind—an impact both scientific and popular. The distinction between the two hemispheres has given rise to pop-psychological theories of all sorts, especially regarding right- and left-brain learning styles or personalities.

What's in a Face?

From time to time over the past fifty years, the neurological literature reports on patients who, having suffered a stroke, could no longer recognize individual human faces, including their own. They could recognize dogs or cats or houses, but not faces. With the advent of brain imaging, it became possible to identify with some precision the areas of the brain that, when damaged, result in problems with face processing.

Face recognition is part of the long-standing debate about how much of the mind/brain operates on special-purpose, "domain-specific" mechanisms. *Domain specific* means that a brain mechanism is dedicated to processing a specific kind of information, such as faces, as opposed to the idea of a general-purpose "domain-general" mechanism, which is capable of operating on any kind of information.

Faces provide an abundance of social information about an individual's gender, age, familiarity, and emotional state and, in some cases, can allow inferences about the intentions or mental states of others. Neuroethologists, having studied across many species the information gained by interpersonal face perception, point out that the primate face has evolved an elaborate system of facial musculature that helps in producing expressive facial movements. What also became clear was the crucial importance of the direction of a gaze. Of course, the eyes have long held a special interest to humans. They have been called "the window of the soul," indicating the richness of information they reveal. Eyes are one of the first points of contact between infants and their mothers.

The critical importance of the eyes to human interactions and human behavior was nicely demonstrated by researchers at Newcastle University in the UK. In the staff common room, they put up an image of eyes on the wall next to a kettle where people made their coffee. They discovered that contributions to the "honesty box" to pay for coffee supplies rose threefold when the eyes were there! None of the forty-eight staff involved was aware of the experiment.[7] University of Washington psychologist Andrew Meltzoff has demonstrated that the behavior of children as young as eighteen months is regulated by the direction of gaze of adults in the room.[8]

Twenty years ago, David Perrett at the University of St. Andrews used single-cell recording techniques to follow up and amplify the observations made by Princeton psychologist Charles Gross that monkeys had brain cells that selectively responded to the sight of monkey and human faces. When Perrett changed the size of the faces, these cells were not affected. But if the individual features of the faces were scrambled, cell responses were markedly reduced. Further research revealed that an important feature of faces for causing these neurons to respond vigorously is the direction of gaze of the eyes and the direction the head is pointing. Perrett also found that the horizontal orientation of the head (looking up or down) had a dramatic effect on the activity of face responsive neurons. All this suggested that one of the key functions of these neurons may be to determine the direction of another's attention. Perrett proposed that the information provided by the eyes, the face, and the movements of the body was each selectively processed by particular groups of neurons, all of which are part of a processing hierarchy for attention direction or socially shared attention.[9]

Another major researcher working on face responsive neurons

is Nancy Kanwisher at MIT. She adds evidence from fMRI of the brains of humans viewing faces to support the results reported by Perrett from single nerve-cell recordings in monkeys. Her work points to what is now called the Fusiform Face Area (part of the medial surface of the temporal lobe) as the place where face-specific processing is localized within the human brain. Kanwisher reviewed the evidence from behavior, neuropsychology, and electrophysiology related to face perception and came down firmly on the side of "domain-specific" mechanisms. Thus, according to Kanwisher, the Fusiform Face Area is specific for the cognitive "domain" of facial processing.[10]

Although there is a clear specificity of mechanisms for face perception in the brain, Kanwisher also notes that this does not rule out the need for plasticity—that is, modification of even "domain-specific" brain functions based on experience and learning. She refers to evidence for the development of face perception in individuals born with dense bilateral cataracts in their eyes. Such people have no pattern vision until their cataracts are surgically corrected between two to six months of age. After such surgery, pattern vision is generally intact, though not completely normal. Surprisingly, these individuals never develop normal face perception. It seems that pattern vision in the first few months of life, particularly experience interacting with other faces, is necessary for the development of normal face processing as an adult. Kanwisher concludes that the "evidence indicates important roles for both genetic factors and specific early experience, in the construction of the Fusiform Face Area."[11] Thus, proper understanding of the nature and extent of localization of function in the brain must also take into account experience-based functional plasticity.

Careful research on face-perception neurons within a particular area of the fusiform gyrus may also provide clues to help us better understand distressing conditions such as autism. Another part of the brain, the inferior temporal gyrus, has been shown to process visual information about objects that do not convey the social and emotional signals found in faces. Using fMRIs, researchers have reported that, when people with autism look at faces, it activates the object-processing areas of the brain. In research participants without autism, the faces activated the fusiform gyrus and the objects, such as cars, activated the inferior temporal gyrus. Individuals with autism appeared to use their object processing center—the inferior temporal gyrus—for both objects (such as cars) and faces. This suggests that some symptoms of autism may come from processing faces as if they are inanimate objects.

Humans (and also monkeys) are social creatures; understanding others' actions is central to survival of both. Christine Keysers and David Perrett have proposed a simple but powerful account of how the monkey brain can learn to understand the actions of others by associating them with self-produced actions, while at the same time discriminating its own actions from those of others.[12] Keysers and Perrett emphasize that understanding even the simplest forms of social cognition involves a complex network of intimately interconnected, but distinct, cortical areas. Since this system also appears to exist in humans, their model can provide a framework for understanding human social perception. Nevertheless, this (presumably) genetically programmed network for social cognition is also modified by environmental interactions. Despite the apparent specialization of the Fusiform Face Area, we must recognize that larger brain networks are also involved. The power of experience to modify this processing, for example, cautions us against drawing simplistic conclusion about the localization of face perception.

Moral Behavior and Personality

In 2000, a schoolteacher began collecting sex magazines and visiting pornographic Web sites, focusing attention on images of children and adolescents. In his own words, "he could not stop himself doing this." When he started making subtle advances to his stepdaughter, his wife called the police. He was arrested for child molestation. He was convicted and underwent a twelve-step rehabilitation program for sexual addicts. The day before his sentencing, he voluntarily went to the hospital to the emergency room with a severe headache. He was distraught and contemplating suicide. The medical staff who examined him said that "he was totally unable to control his impulses" and "he had propositioned the nurses." An MRI scan was taken of his brain and revealed an egg-sized tumor pressing on his right frontal lobe. The frontal lobe tumor was removed. His lewd behavior and pedophilia faded away. A year later, the tumor partially grew back, and the man started once again to collect pornography. A further operation was undertaken to remove the regrowing tumor and his urges again subsided.[13]

There was widespread comment on this case. A neurologist said that "he saw people with brain tumors who would lie, damage property, and in extreme rare cases, commit murder." He further commented, "The individuals simply lose the ability to control impulses or anticipate the consequences of choices." A psychiatrist specializing in behavioral changes associated with brain disorders and who had studied the way in which brain tumors can affect a person's behavior, provocatively commented, "This tells us something about being human, doesn't it? . . . If one's actions are governed by how well the brain is working does it mean we have less free will than we think?"[14]

All these specialists know that human behavior is governed by complex interactions in the brain. Many neuroscientists believe that "executive processes" in behavior—making decisions with major consequences—are dependent upon the normal functioning of systems within, and/or linked to, the frontal lobes. The frontal lobes are regarded as the most highly evolved area of the brain. Tumors in this area can squeeze enough blood from the region to effectively put it to sleep, thus dulling the person's judgment in a way similar to drinking too much alcohol. However, only in very rare cases will the tumor turn the person to violence or deviant behavior.

The dramatic changes, and then reversal, in the teacher's behavior provide a vivid illustration of how our moral behavior is embodied in our physical make-up. Similarly dramatic effects have been on record for a long time in the case of Phineas Gage, a case known well by every student of neurology and neuropsychology. Gage's frontal lobes were damaged in an accident, the result of which was that his behavior was permanently changed for the worse. From being a reliable industrious pillar of society, he became dissolute, capricious, and irresponsible. As primatologist Frans de Waal has written of Gage and other such patients, "It's as if the moral compass of these people has been demagnetized, causing it to spin out of control. What this incident teaches us is that conscience is not some disembodied concept that can be understood only on the basis of culture and religion."[15] Morality, he claimed, is as firmly grounded in neurobiology as anything else we do or are.

Such dramatic cases are easily oversimplified. Media reports can spread the impression that specific parts of the brain completely control certain behavior. Narrowly speaking, this can be true. For example, damage to a small area of the cortex serving vision (called "V4") can strip color from the vision, leaving a visual world limited to shades of grays. It is only natural to describe V4 as a "color area." But it is important to remember that this should not imply that this area functions in isolation to give rise to color vision: it is a necessary but not a sufficient area.

Most often in the waking brain, very large numbers of small cortical regions work in parallel on their specialized tasks. Thus, while the dramatic changes observed in a patient like Phineas Gage are often described as part of the "frontal-lobe syndrome," aspects of the same frontal syndrome can also appear as a consequence of damage to a much lower part of the brain known as the pedunculopontine tegmental nucleus. Much of the data regarding this lower brain nucleus has been gathered from lesion studies in rats, but damage to similar areas in humans may produce similar results. Supporting such a view further is the work of Cambridge psychologist Trevor Robbins and his group who have examined frontal-lobe-like deficits in many types of neurological patients, including a group with progressive supranuclear palsy—a disorder caused by degeneration of subcortical motor nuclei.[16] These patients did poorly on tests of their frontal-lobe function. Philip Winn, a psychologist at St. Andrews University, notes that "often no obvious or extensive damage to the frontal lobes can be seen in patients who display many frontal lobe deficits."[17]

Before we leave this review of links between our brains and our capacity for moral behavior, we should reflect on one more recent study that seems out of the ordinary. Conducted by C. B. Gensch and colleagues, this study showed that other sorts of physical changes, not involving damage to neural structures, can also affect behavior. They reported that the reduction in a person's diet of vitamins, minerals, and fatty acids can also lead to increased antisocial behavior.[18]

We began this chapter with ideas about a "self," "mind," or "soul" that seems to be inside of us, controlling our bodies. One more example reminds us of this common intuition. If you put on stereo headphones and listen to your favorite singer, then ask yourself, "Where does the singer I am listening to seem to be?" The obvious answer based on what you are *experiencing* is, "The singer is in the middle of my head." The headphones put the sound right between the ears, so that is where the singer seems to be. Of course, things are not always what they *seem*.

In respect to mental activity, and the subjective experience of an inner "me," we hope to have shown that the origins are not what they seem. Our subjective mental life is not separable from the activity of our physical bodies. Each of us seems to have within us a stream of feelings, images, and inner talk that we experience as transcending our body. But all of these phenomena come about by the operation of neural systems. For example, my inner talk is the subjective experience of off-line motor speech systems running scenarios and emulations of physically speaking. I experience inner speech in much the same way as I experience my own speaking out loud—as inside my head. In the case of the split-brain patient, we are confronted with the fact that we only experience the world as unified (rather than two distinct worlds, one in each cerebral hemisphere) due to neural activity traveling back and forth across the pathway know as the corpus callosum.

We have seen that one argument for the physical embodiment of these psychological and mental experiences is the occurrence of predictable mental defects when particular brain areas are damaged. Another argument is the degree to which particular forms of mental processing are consistently accompanied by activity in localized brain areas. Particular brain areas are highly active, for example, during speaking or hearing language, perceiving faces, and contemplating the consequences (particularly the moral consequences) of our behavior.

However, in addition to this take-home message about the embodiment of the mental life, we must remember how the phrenologists of the past—and their modern counterparts—have tended to become too literal about the localization of mental properties in particular brain regions. This is the slippery slope toward the so-called "God module," an attempt to localize religious experiences in specific brain regions. We have countered this simplistic notion of localization by showing that areas with "domain-specificity" are nevertheless nested in larger, more complex, and looping networks that contribute important forms of information analysis. In addition, all cortical areas of the brain develop their particular processing characteristics under the influence of learning, particularly during early life development.

As mentioned earlier, comparative psychology (also called evolutionary psychology) has looked at the brains of many species, helping to gather further evidence of links between mind and brain. Now we turn to research that compares apes and humans— for some, perhaps, the most controversial type of brain science. The topic fascinates, for it raises ultimate questions about our religious beliefs and moral choices, our freedom and responsibility, and in what sense human beings are truly "unique" in the animal kingdom.

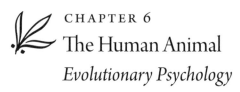

CHAPTER 6

The Human Animal
Evolutionary Psychology

IT IS HARD to avoid popular headlines today about the new "evolutionary psychology," which seemingly purports to explain the evolutionary origins of every kind of human behavior. Such popular reports—on everything from courtship between men and women to our responses to marketing—splash across the covers of *Time* and *Der Spiegel* magazines, not to mention scientific journals such as *Science* and *Nature*. This approach has also gained notoriety, and stirred controversy, under the name sociobiology.

The appeal relates to how evolution tries to show how human beings, on the one hand, are similar to animals (and even ant colonies!) but, on the other, are somehow unique—we emerged from other species with a whole range of specialized and "superior" abilities. Our relationship to the various species of nonhuman primates brings this topic closest to home. This discussion has major implications for both humanist and religious views about human nature. Overall, as research advances, lines that formerly had seemed to divide animals and humans now become increasingly blurred, making the question of human uniqueness ever more problematic.

What is today called "evolutionary psychology" used to be labeled "comparative psychology." It has an illustrious history in psychology's development. An important assumption in comparative psychology was voiced at the beginning of the twentieth century by Lloyd Morgan, the British scientist. Morgan's famous canon proposed that "in no case may we interpret an action as the outcome of a higher psychical faculty if it can be interpreted as the outcome of one which stands lower in the psychological scale."[1]

Early comparative psychology focused on finding links between changes in sensory processes and learning as one moves up the phylogenetic tree of evolution. This, in turn, led to attempts to link the increasing complexity of the brain and central nervous system with more elaborate behaviors and learning capacities. Soon enough, the findings of ethologists such as Conrad Lorenz and Nikolaas Tinbergen revealed the fallacy of believing that increased complexity of the nervous system always meant increasing complexity of learning capacity and social behavior. Some of the animals with the simplest nervous systems showed remarkably complex forms of social behavior—consider, for example, the ants and the bees.

Evolutionary psychology bases its study of human thinking and behavior on the evolutionary principles of natural selection. Accordingly, it presumes that natural selection favored genes that engendered our ancestor with behaviors and brain-processing systems that solved survival problems, thus contributing to the spread of their genes. In 1992, John Tooby and Leda Cosmides defined evolutionary psychology as "psychology informed by the fact that the inherited structure of the human mind is a product of evolutionary processes."[2] Thus, the main focus of research in evolutionary psychology is the question of how humans came to be the special animal that we seem to be.

According to evolutionary psychologist Richard Byrne, some of the central questions in this field are: When did a particular cognitive trait enter the human lineage? What was the trait's original adaptive function? Has it been retained for the same reason, or is it now valuable for some different purpose? Furthermore, what is the cognitive basis for the behavioral trait, and how does its organization relate to other mental capacities?[3]

In discussions of comparative and evolutionary psychology, anthropomorphism figures large. As a result, popular reporting easily gives the impression that it is unproblematic to interpret the behavior of animals closest to us on the evolutionary scale based on our human experience. Frans de Waal comments:

> This use of anthropomorphism as a means to get at the truth, rather than an end in itself, sets its use in science apart from use by the lay person. . . . The ultimate goal of the scientist is emphatically not to arrive at the most satisfactory projection of human feelings onto the animal, but rather at testable ideas and replicable observations. Thus, anthropomorphism serves the same exploratory function as that of intuition in all science, from mathematics to medicine.[4]

To illustrate some of the hottest research questions in contemporary evolutionary psychology, we shall review four research topics: (1) language, (2) "theory of mind" and mirror-neurons, (3) social intelligence, and (4) altruistic-looking behavior in animals. These topics will also suggest how this research is relevant to wider issues of understanding the nature of human uniqueness and how these issues prompt a reexamination of some of our religious views of our human nature.

LANGUAGE

Perhaps the greatest evolutionary leap between the mental capacities of the most intelligent nonhuman primates and that of human beings lies in the use of language. However, the apparent size of the chasm traversed has been reduced by the extensive work done over the last twenty years in attempting to teach great apes a language system. The research on ape language has revealed much not previously known about the capacity of apes to communicate using an abstract system of symbols or gestures (including the ability of some to understand human speech). While the linguistic performance of apes has clear limitations, much can be learned about the evolutionary roots of language by studying nonhuman primates.

The natural signaling systems that apes use in the wild are basically closed systems composed of a finite number of basic vocal expressions. These primarily communicate emotional states elicited by a few types of environmental stimuli. Such complexity as exists in the primate's natural signaling system results from gradations and modulations of this small number of basic signal types (not unlike emotional prosody in human language). Thus, apes in the wild cannot be considered to have developed language.

Explicit attempts to teach expanded, abstract communication systems to apes have met with some success. Most of these experiments have involved attempts to teach chimpanzees to communicate with a human being using abstract symbols or tokens or using the gestures of American Sign Language. However, the meaning of this research with respect to a language system (versus rote learning) has been controversial. Apes clearly show the intent of communicating with an abstract system. They have mastered a limited multiword vocabulary and demonstrated an ability to use multiword expressions (two to six words at most) that appear to make sense. Still, we are not sure whether apes instructed in this kind of abstract communication truly possess a structured, rule-governed grammar. Many linguists argue that they have been taught a more sophisticated signaling system, but hardly a language.

Most of the early attempts to teach a language system to chimpanzees began with adult animals. More recent work suggests that chimps raised from infancy in a language-rich environment (more like the experience of human children) obtain a higher level of ability. In their work *Kanzi: The Ape at the Brink of the Human Mind* (1994), American primatologists Sue Savage-Rumbaugh and Roger Levin describe the remarkable language capacity of a bonobo (or pygmy chimpanzee) named Kanzi. As an infant, Kanzi was a passive participant in unsuccessful attempts to teach language to his mother. When finally allowed to express himself via the language system that was being taught to his mother, Kanzi seemed to know spontaneously how to communicate with the symbols and to have developed an unusual (for a chimpanzee) general language processing capacity. Most remarkable was Kanzi's grasp of spoken English. Kanzi eventually was capable of understanding a wide variety of spoken sentence types (thirteen in all), including sentences with embedded phrases. Kanzi responded correctly on 74 percent of 660 novel sentences, including some recognition of semantics carried by word order. This capacity was considered roughly comparable to that of a normal two-and-a-half-year-old human.

In 2007, a report from a meeting on "The Mind of the Chimpanzee" suggested that there is now strong evidence that language started with gesturing. Amy Pollick and Frans de Waal carefully studied four groups of apes living in captivity. Two of the groups were chimpanzees and two were bonobos (pygmy chimpanzees). They videotaped their behavior for hundreds of hours over more than a year. They concentrated on recording facial and vocal expressions, hand and foot gestures, and the behavioral context in which these expressions and gestures took place.[5]

Their hypothesis was that the meaning of facial expressions is hardwired by evolution, whereas the meaning of gestures is learned and, to some extent, arbitrary. The researchers found that facial expressions always occurred in the same contexts in different groups and different species. This was not true for gestures, however. Half of the routine gestures had completely different meanings in the two species. Even within a single group, the meaning of a gesture varied with the context. Gesturing, it seems, is a likely forerunner of language: it is comprised of more arbitrary links between the physical signal and its meaning. In this context, it is worth remembering that gesture remains a crucial part of human language— just watch anyone walking along using a mobile phone! Evolution does not come up with complicated new structures or capacities in a single leap but builds them up step-by-step. Pollick and de Waal believe that the capacity for speech is built on mental attributes that were acquired millions of years ago when the ancestors of apes and humans began to gesture meaningfully at each other.

Another theory suggests that the key component of language ability is focused in the left hemisphere of the human brain and in a specific gene called protocadhedrinXY.[6] This gene, so it is claimed, can be said to define our species. On this view, the emergence of *Homo sapiens* was not a gradual or continuous process; instead, there is the possibility that, 100,000 to 150,000 years ago, a relatively abrupt jump gave rise to our species. The jury is certainly still out on judging this recent proposal.

Impressed as we are by Kanzi, such outcomes do not emerge spontaneously. They depend on support from a human linguistic community. Unlike Kanzi, apes in the wild develop no more than a contextually and emotionally modulated set of vocal signals, and they acquire some communicative gestures. It takes human instructors to teach adolescent or adult apes to use symbols or gestures with anything like linguistic properties. But again, the fact of Kanzi is an amazing finding: young chimpanzees extensively exposed to human language can understand it in ways not measurably different from a normal two-and-a-half-year-old human. After the point, of course, young human children (three years old) move rapidly ahead with a far more sophisticated expressive grammar and much greater linguistic creativity.

THEORY OF MIND

For any species, dealing with other members is a challenge for which evolution has produced a number of specialized abilities. In primates, a set of highly complex cognitive abilities is the very key to a successful social life. We humans have an irresistible tendency, for example, to translate our understanding of the behavior of others into an assumption about their mental states. We represent what people are doing in terms of what we believe they want and of what we believe they know and do not know. It is this ability that has come to be known in cognitive science as "theory of mind." Because we cannot see what is in a person's mind, we make a reasonable inference (theories) about that mind by what the person does or says. As far back as 1978, David Premack and Guy Woodruff described animals that had the ability to understand the mind of another, becoming the first to refer to this ability as a "theory of mind."[7] Andrew Whiten and Richard Byrne (two leaders in the field of evolutionary psychology) provide a useful definition:

> Having a theory of mind or being able to mind-read concerns the ability of an individual to respond differentially, according to assumptions about the beliefs and desires of another individual, rather than in direct response to the others' overt behavior.[8]

Comparative and evolutionary psychology both ask the same question: do nonhuman primates represent to themselves the behavior of other members of their species in a similar mentalistic way? In the absence of language, the task of studying this form of mind reading in animals is difficult. Developmental psychologists, for example, use language to study what children know about the beliefs of others. But in the absence of language, what methods are available to primatologists?

Basic to a theory of mind is the ability, first, to read the focus of another's attention and, second, to comprehend the intentions signaled by the actions of another. These basic forms are amenable to study in primates. Inferring the focus of attention of another has been studied extensively in chimpanzees and is reported in the literature on deception—what is called "Machiavellian intelligence."[9] The capacity of reading another individual's intentions begins in children at age two-and-a-half, and is fairly well developed by age four. As far as we know, a primate's ability to read intentions never gets to the level of the four-year-old human. Similarly, there is no evidence in nonhuman primates of understanding false beliefs–the litmus test for the presence of a theory of mind in human children.

Most of the evidence for a theory of mind in primates has come from observational studies and only recently (and to a limited extent) from experiments. Byrne and Whiten, in field observations of primates, described in their two volumes on *Machiavellian Intelligence* (1988, 1997) frequently witnessed behaviors of the following kind: They see a female baboon interested in a young male; however, the dominant male would promptly intervene if he saw them doing things like grooming each other, the sort of exchanges that forge bonds among baboons. So, on this particular occasion, a deceptive rendezvous seems to unfold.

It begins when the young male moves behind a rock so he is not visible to the dominant male. The female moves herself slowly but steadily toward the rock, seemingly just looking at the details of the grass and the ground. Eventually, she moves behind the rock, but she does this in a way that the upper part of her body can still be seen from the other side. At the same time, she starts grooming the completely hidden young male, who remains invisible to the dominant male. So the dominant male can't see the offending action, but he can see where the female is, and the female, at the same time, can watch the movements of the dominant male. With respect to a theory of mind, the important questions are: Do the young male and female understand how clever they are being? Are they acting "according to a plan" to conceal their offending actions? Given that the female makes herself visible, is she somehow reckoning that the dominant male will mistakenly think she is alone behind the rock?

Further links of evolutionary psychology with social neuroscience have been made by those who argue that the capacity for certain forms of deception in some nonhuman primates (which looks like mind reading in humans) has resulted from a rapid evolutionary increase in neocortical volume. They point out that there is a direct relationship between neocortical volume and amount of such "clever-looking" behaviors. This relationship with neocortical volume also applies to deception, innovation, and tool use. Richard Byrne has written:

> Quite what benefits a large neo-cortex brings—the underlying cognitive basis of monkey and ape social sophistication—is not straightforward to answer. It is tempting, but may be utterly wrong, to assume that an animal that works over many months to build-up a friendly relationship has some idea of the effect its behavior is having on the mind of the other.... We assume the agent realizes that by producing a false belief in his victim may risk losing a friend or gaining an enemy. The alternative is a more prosaic mixture of genetic predisposition and rapid learning—and often this is more likely.[10]

The views held by evolutionary psychologists can change rapidly. This is illustrated by the research on theory of mind. It used to be argued that only humans have a "theory of mind." Up until 2000, Michael Tomasello believed that the observational data reported by Byrne and Whiten claiming to show forms of rudimentary "mind reading" in chimpanzees were not convincing evidence that nonhuman primates have a theory of mind.[11] Today, Tomasello, on the basis of his own laboratory studies, is convinced that his earlier views are wrong and in need of revision. In 2003, he wrote:

> In our 1997 book *Primate Cognition* we reviewed all the available evidence and concluded that nonhuman primates understand much about behavior of conspecifics but nothing about their psychological states, [but] . . . in the last five years new data have emerged that require modification of this hypothesis. The form that a new hypothesis should take is not entirely clear, but we are now convinced that at least some nonhuman primates—

the research is mainly on chimpanzees—do understand at least some psychological states in others. . . . For the moment we feel safe in asserting that chimpanzees can understand some psychological states in others, the question is only which ones and to what extent.[12]

The developmental psychologist Simon Baron-Cohen has suggested that autism demonstrates what human life would be like without a "theory of mind." He says that the kind of deceptive behavior documented in nonhuman primates is no trivial achievement. The deceiver needs to have the mental equipment to juggle different representations of reality. He further notes that the neurological condition that leads to difficulties in socializing, in chatting with others, also leads to difficulties in recognizing when someone might be deceiving them, and that nicely sums up some of the major problems faced by people with autism.

Baron-Cohen comments:

> Many children with autism are perplexed by why someone would even want to deceive others, why someone would think about fiction or pretence. They have no difficulty with fact (what he calls version 1 of reality) and can tell you easily if something is true or false ("Is the moon made of rocks? Yes! Is the moon made of cheese? No!"). . . . They may be puzzled by version 2 of reality that, "John believes the moon is made of cheese." Why should a person believe something that is untrue?[13]

In this sense, Cohen believes such children show some degree of "mindblindness." They do not have a fully developed theory of mind. As he explains further:

> Even the higher functioning children on the autistic spectrum, such as those with Asperger's syndrome,

show delays in the development of mind-reading ability. This neurological (and ultimately genetic) set of conditions can leave the person with autism or Asperger's syndrome prey to deception and exploitation.[14]

In a word, this new kind of research in evolutionary psychology may provide medical insights into some extremely trying neurological conditions that up to now have been very difficult to fathom.

Mind Reading: The Mirror Neuron Story

If an actual mechanism for the so-called mind-reading behavior of primates could be found, it would be a natural bridge between neuroscience, evolutionary psychology, and social cognition. Some have heralded such a discovery in a neural substrate, or cell tissue, called the mirror neuron.

The mirror neuron story began twenty years ago when Italian neurophysiologist Giacomo Rizzolatti and his colleagues reported the discovery of neurons in the frontal lobes of the brains of monkeys, which possessed functional properties not previously observed.[15] The unusual property of these cells was that they were active not only when a monkey initiated a particular action but also when the animal observed another monkey initiating and carrying out the same action. For this reason, they were labeled by some as the "monkey-see-monkey-do" cells. These unusual neurons did not respond when the monkey was merely presented with a conventional visual stimulus. Rather, they were activated only when the monkey saw another individual (whether the human experimenter or another monkey) making a goal-directed action with a hand or mouth.

Vittorio Gallese (a collaborator with Rizzolatti in the study of mirror neurons) speculated that a primary and important role of mirror neurons is that they underlie the process of "mind reading," or are at least a precursor to such a process.[16] The potential importance of this work on mirror neurons for understanding social cognition was also recognized by V. S. Ramachandran (a research neurologist at the University of California, San Diego). He wrote, "I predict that mirror neurons will do for psychology what DNA did for biology"—a truly bold and far-reaching suggestion.[17] Ramachandran believes that understanding the role of these cells may give us a deeper insight into how we assign intentions and beliefs to other inhabitants of our social world. Thus, the discovery and description of the responses of these important neurons represents the convergence of state-of-the-art research in neuroscience, evolutionary biology, and psychology.

Functional brain imaging has made it possible to examine the neural substrates of movement-production, perception of action, and imagery in humans. Results indicate that witnessing the hand movements of another person activates the prefrontal cortex in the homologous area where mirror neurons were found in the monkey. Thus, activity in this area of the human brain is believed to constitute the neural basis for imitating the actions of others, as well as inferring the intentions of those actions (that is to say, "mind reading"). As you might expect, there is great debate among active workers in this field about what constitutes true imitation, what constitutes mind reading, and what might be the relationship between data from brain imaging in humans and direct nerve-cell recordings in primates.

SOCIAL INTELLIGENCE

In their 1988 book *Machiavellian Intelligence*, Byrne and Whiten looked at the complexities of the social life of our ancestors as a possible route to understanding the development of our distinctive abilities. In 1997, in a second volume under the same title, they extended their findings and argued that intelligence began in social manipulation, deceit, and cunning cooperation. Humankind is, of course, at the apex of this evolutionary development of social intelligence. Thus, Whiten further argues that what differentiates human society from chimpanzee society is the level of cognitive sophistication at which social integration and interaction occurs. Whiten calls this distinguishing feature a "deep social mind" and further claims that

> humans are more social—more deeply social—than any other species on earth, our closest primate relatives not excepted. . . . by "deep" I am referring to a special degree of cognitive and mental penetration between individuals.[18]

Careful observations in the wild and detailed testing in captivity have both produced a wealth of new data on chimpanzee social behavior, so much so, in fact, that Whiten recalls that, fifty years ago, when so little was known, the current findings about a complex chimpanzee society could have not been imagined. This view is endorsed by de Waal, who points out that, even a decade ago, there was no firm consensus on chimpanzee society. Today, there is little debate. Nevertheless, in evaluating the evidence for sophisticated social behavior in animals, we should follow Byrne's warning of the dangers of drawing inferences from field observations alone:

> Researchers have to be very cautious, then, in attributing to non-human primates the ability to understand social behavior or how things work in the mechanistic way of adult humans. Rapid learning in social circumstances, a good memory for individuals and their different characteristics, and some simple genetic tendencies are capable of explaining much that has impressed observers as intelligent in simian primates.[19]

If humans have a "deep social mind" compared to a chimpanzee, what is it in brain structure that might account for this difference? Recent research has proposed that the critical element is an enhancement in neural wiring—namely, a proliferation of Von Economo neurons. These neurons are very large neurons that have very long axons projecting throughout much of the cerebral cortex. The origin of Von Economo neurons is the limbic cortex—specifically, the anterior cingulate gyrus and insula of the cortex. The insular cortex receives information about the state of the body (that is, visceral/autonomic information, including feedback from bodily responses that would occur in emotions). The anterior cingulate cortex consistently shows activity when an individual is making decisions in the social or moral domain and during the experience of social emotions. Under neuroimaging, both the anterior cingulate cortex and the insula showed marked activity during states of empathy, shame, trust, and humor, as well as during detection of the mental and emotional states and during moral decision making.

According to the theory of Caltech neuroscientists John Allman, Patrick Hof, and their colleagues, the experience of bodily emotions converges on the anterior cingulate and insular cortex, which spread this information through the cortex by way of the Von Economo neurons. This process informs the cognitive functions of these emotional states.[20] This final integration of bodily states with higher cognition allows the human brain to comprehend emotion itself, thus signaling to a person the social significance of actions and perceptions.

The Von Economo neurons are important in any discussion about the "deep social mind" of humanity because they are relatively unique to the human brain. This type of neuron is found in great abundance in the adult human brain and in the brain of a four-year-old child, but they are few in number in newborn human infants and in apes and entirely nonexistent in lower primates.[21] It is also of interest that these neurons have been found to be about 30 percent more numerous in the right hemisphere of the human brain, often thought to be particularly involved in the processing of emotional information.[22]

Evolutionary psychology has tended to reject any theoretical efforts to separate cognitive capacities (like language) from social capacities and experiences because it views these two domains as integrated in mutually reinforcing ways, finally making the complexity of the human being unprecedented compared to monkeys and great apes. Social interactions, therefore, seem to be crucial in shaping human behavior and priming the appearance of the highest and most complex cognitive skills, including language.

ALTRUISTIC BEHAVIOR IN ANIMALS

Over the past three decades, researchers have increasingly observed that some animal behaviors, if seen in humans, might be called moral or altruistic. "Aiding others at a cost or risk to oneself is widespread in the animal world," according to primatologist de Waal."[23] Attempts to understand such "altruistic" behavior had been closely linked to a genecentric sociobiology. According to this view, genes favor their own replication: a gene is successful if it produces a trait that, in turn, promotes the continuance of the gene. To describe this idea of genetic self-promotion, the Oxford zoologist Richard Dawkins introduced the psychological term *selfish* in the title of his book *The Selfish Gene*. What might normally be called a generous act in common language, such as bringing home food, now was interpreted as actually "selfish" from the gene's perspective.

As the original meaning of the words *from the gene's perspec*tive were forgotten and then discarded, we now hear a constant discussion in biology about how *all* behavior is selfish. Obviously, however, genes have neither a self nor emotions to make them selfish. The phrase is simply a metaphor. Nevertheless, when a metaphor is repeated often enough—even in science—it can assume an aura of literal truth. Dawkins himself had cautioned against going too far with his anthropomorphic talk about a selfish gene, but to little effect. To redress this distortion, de Waal and other biologists are trying to separate the "selfish" metaphor from the actual scientific findings that show remarkable social behaviors in animals.

Once this confusion is cleared up, evolutionary theory can use the genetic make-up of the organism to try to explain the evolution of a capacity of aid to others. That genetic explanation comes in two general ways:

1. Genes favoring altruism can spread in future generations if the costs of the genetically related altruistic behavior to the altruists' personal reproductive success are outweighed by the benefits in reproductive success of the altruists' relatives carrying copies of the same genes. This is termed *kin selection*.

2. Genes favoring altruism could also spread if the altruism is sufficiently reciprocated (*reciprocal altruism*)—that is to say, the benefit bestowed by the altruist on another is received back in kind.

As regards kin selection, examples are widespread in the animal kingdom. Some of its most extreme forms are found, as one might expect, in those odd species where individuals in the colony are unusually highly related to each other. For example, in social insects like bees and ants, the genetic relatedness of workers to each other and to the queen is three-quarters (whereas the maximum found in mammals is one-half, based on relations between a parent and child and between siblings). This is taken to explain why sterile castes of workers evolved in ants and bees; these workers are totally altruistic, spending their whole lives giving food for the "good of the group" (or the good of the queen, who is the only one to reproduce directly). One of the most graphic examples is "honey-pot" worker ants, who do nothing but hang from the ceiling of the ant colony, acting as receptacles or storage jars for honey, which some workers fill them with and which the colony draws on when needed. At the individual ant level, that is self-sacrifice!

Examples of reciprocal altruism appear to be much rarer. Apart from human beings, there are only a handful of examples. A classic example is the vampire bat. Vampire bats are in real danger of starving if they should fail to get their blood meal on a particular evening. However, if this happens, they are fed back in their colony by an unrelated nest mate, to whom they are likely to repay the favor on another night.

We should not assume, however, that, because two behaviors appear to be similar (for example, in animals and humans), therefore, the underlying behavioral mechanisms are similar or identical. In high-tech laboratories, we can now reproduce aspects of human and animal behavior in robots. Still, no one suggests that the underlying mechanisms producing those behaviors are the same. They may share some common features but, when it comes to questions of motivation, conscious awareness, and goal-directed behavior, the two may be miles apart. Likewise, because we can observe self-giving, self-sacrificing behavior in different evolutionary phyla, that tells us nothing about the underlying mechanisms involved. How, for example, could a behavior be "self-giving" if there is no awareness of "self"?

There are some compelling (but anecdotal) examples of self-giving behavior in nonhuman primates. Field-working primatologist Jane Goodall describes unusual chimpanzee behaviors that are not done by all chimpanzees or even by particular chimpanzees routinely. This includes a female helping her mother, even though the mother is unlikely to help the daughter in return or reproduce their genes again. Such anecdotal observations are scientifically problematic, but they certainly are different from the ant cases already mentioned. Here we have an unusual episode in which the female recognized her mother as in need of help and worked out a way to help her.

As we already emphasized, self-giving behaviors in different animals do not tells us the roots of those behaviors. Self-giving may occur, for example, with or without self-awareness. We also have very persuasive arguments that self-giving and self-limiting behavior in organisms developed during a long evolutionary history and eventually emerged in nonhuman primates. That evolutionary viewpoint does not make the behavior any less worthy, nor does it argue that humans are "nothing but" complex primates. Emotions are easily stirred whenever someone notes the similarity between human and nonhuman primate behavior. Some of these behaviors are clearly related. But the idea that humans are "nothing but" glorified apes ignores the distinctiveness of the ethical, moral, and religious aspects of human cognition and behavior.

This warning against reductionism is brought out in de Waal's 1996 book *Good Natured*, which tells us that

> even if animals other than ourselves act in ways tantamount to moral behavior, their behavior does not necessarily rest on deliberations of the kind we engage in. It is hard to believe that animals weigh their own interests against the rights of others, that they develop a view of the greater good of society, or that they feel lifelong guilt about something they should not have done.... To communicate intentions and feelings is one thing; and to clarify what is right, and why, and what is wrong, and why, is quite something else. Animals are not moral philosophers.[24]

Regarding that moral sense, he also writes that "the fact that the human moral sense goes so far back in evolutionary history that other species show signs of it, plants morality firmly near to the centre of our much maligned nature." He adds that "humankind's uniqueness is embodied in a suite of features that include ethical behavior and religious beliefs."[25]

Other leading evolutionary psychologists, who have no religious axe to grind, also criticize the excessive enthusiasm to equating nonhuman primates and humans, warning that such exaggeration can jeopardize the scientific work. Richard Byrne, in commenting on a reported trend for human stepfathers to murder their partner's babies under three years old, warned against forcing such findings among animals into assumptions about so-called evolutionary stable strategies among humans:

> These [behaviors] are not carefully thought out by beasts; and nor are any genes really selfish or altruistic, they are no more than pieces of DNA molecules; nor is an understanding of kinship likely to be remotely similar to our own. [Concepts like murder and altruism] are human applied labels based on the superficial appearance of the actions of individual animals whose behavior is partially governed by genes.... Natural selection is a mechanistic process and thus morally neutral; discovering a genetic influence on murder does not condone it.... Human social behavior is [by contrast] influenced by our culture and our extensive information transmission by spoken and written language in ways not well described by biology.[26]

HUMAN DISTINCTIVENESS: SEARCH FOR THE QUANTUM LEAP

Such comparisons between humans and other species have not stopped the search for the "quantum leap," or as some say "phase change," that was necessary to make humans so different from animals. This is a scientific puzzle that will occupy us for many years to come. There are serious scientific issues to be addressed here, and it may be tempting, in a search for human uniqueness, to seize upon a particular human capacity (such as "mind reading") as one way of uniquely separating off humans from nonhumans. At the same time, when similarities between the behavior of humans and some nonhuman primates are identified, there will be the temptation to say that humans are "nothing but" unusually complex primates.

For most people, however, probably the very first obstacle in this scientific discussion is their feeling that it is demeaning, and even offensive, to compare humans directly with apes. They might be given the wise counsel that, in fact, we can gain much self-knowledge in this comparison. Still, that does not always clear away the emotional obstacles. Perhaps the best way to approach the comparison of ourselves and animals is first to ask, "Is there a difference in kind or merely a difference in degree?" In the seventeenth century, the French mathematician Blaise Pascal approached this type of question by discussing it from a theological point of view:

> It is dangerous to show a man too clearly how much alike he is to the beasts without showing him his greatness. It is also dangerous to show him too clearly his greatness without his lowliness. It is still more dangerous to leave him in ignorance of both.[27]

This discussion also can be confused by the term *uniqueness*, which has several dimensions. Animals of each phylum are unique. Each has properties and abilities none others do. Birds can fly and we cannot (at least unaided). For the religious person who might worry about these modern comparisons of humans and animals, it is helpful to know that evolutionary psychology, as a science, has nothing at stake in the religious question of human uniqueness. The science does not draw a theological conclusion, even though individual psychologists, based on their personal beliefs, may probe these theological questions.

As a science, evolutionary psychology simply hopes that the study of animal behavior will help us detect possible beginnings of language and our own ability to possess a theory of mind, and see the seeds of human culture in chimpanzee societies. We can pursue this research carefully and still avoid the temptation to adopt unjustified implications for human behavior that we glean from observing other animals.

One useful analogy for explaining the remarkable cognitive and social gap between nonhuman and human primates is that of a "phase change," a concept used in physics. This kind of change occurs when the same basic materials (in our case, having a basic animal brain system) suddenly or gradually exhibits new properties. In physics, oxygen and hydrogen in appropriate proportions and under specific conditions become a liquid with different properties from gases. In another example, the physicist and theologian John Polkinghorne recounts how the seeming irrationality of the superconductivity state made sense only when it was realized that

> there was a higher rationality than that known in the everyday world of Ohm. After more than 50 years of theoretical effort, an understanding of current flow in metals was found which subsumed both ordinary conduction and superconductivity into a single theory. The different behaviors correspond to different regimes, characterized by different organizations of the states of motion of electrons in the metal. One regime changes into the other by phase change (as the physicists call it) at the critical temperature.[28]

Despite this obvious gap between the social and mental life of humans and other animals, evolutionary psychology has produced evidence that animals can indeed think as some level. Such behaviors in humans would be typically described as imagination, inventiveness, and means-end reasoning. In the case of "mind reading," evolutionary psychology and neuroscience have developed explanations for how this emerged even in animals. As a result of this research into the thinking powers of the brain, it has become difficult to draw a clear demarcation between the mental abilities of nonhuman primates and humans.

This fuzzy boundary between humans and animals should not really bother a religious outlook, since the important aspects of human uniqueness are based on theological presuppositions, not on neurobiological observations. At the same time, humans are clearly unique by way of their explosive development of learning, philosophy, literature, music, art, science, and so on. What needs to be said about animals is only this: they do show reasoning and thinking abilities. While this ability is rudimentary, it overlaps with similar abilities in developing human children. At the most, therefore, scientific research has made it difficult to use the marks of thinking or reasoning as the sole anchor to claim that humans are created in the image of God.

Some Christians may be concerned about this narrowing of the gap between ourselves and some nonhuman primates. For our part, we believe that there are no great issues at stake in this research. As the quotes above demonstrate, the careful scholars and workers in this field also are dismayed by the popular exaggerations in the media. A Christian can be enthusiastically open-minded about developments in evolutionary psychology—not gullible, but discerning, and glimpsing fresh pointers to the greatness of the Creator in the wonders of his creation. This is another area of science where we may exercise stewardship by engaging in new research on such distressing mental conditions as autism and, in this way, show care and compassion.

The course of creation has been such that the qualities of self-giving and self-limiting behavior, built upon neural substrates, may be traced out, coming to full flower in humankind. This is not to say that such behavior is genetically determined. Its expression increases and multiplies moment by moment, depending on personal choices and arguably on the catalytic effect of living in a self-giving community. Again, constant vigilance is called for to avoid slipping into sloppy thinking that assumes that similarities in overt behavior demonstrate identical mechanisms for those behaviors.

Speaking personally, from within our shared Christian tradition, we do not find it necessary to deny the emergence of elements of altruistic or self-giving behavior in nonhuman primates in order for us to affirm the reality of what is called *agape* love, seen uniquely in the self-giving and self-emptying of Jesus Christ. The self-giving of Christ was unique, and it is by faith that we affirm that the ultimate act of Christ's self-giving, by its nature, sets him and it apart from all others.

CHAPTER 7
The Neuroscience of Religiousness

MOST OF US have seen people who have lost cognitive abilities after suffering a neurological disease or brain disorder. For some of these cases, the loss originated in congenital brain damage. Other people face the loss later in life, either by suffering a traumatic brain injury or a progressive neurological disorder like Alzheimer's and Parkinson's diseases. These everyday stories confirm what the contemporary research tells us: without the intactness of the physical body and brain, people lose qualities of reasoning, memory, language, recognition of faces, "mind reading," and even personality.

In the context of illness, these links between the body and mind do not surprise us. What about religion, however? Should we be surprised at what neuroscience is discovering about religiousness, moral judgments, and social relationships? Based on the ubiquity of religion, spirituality, and mysticism in human experience, the human being has been called the "religious species," or *Homo religio*. We have been more commonly called *Homo sapiens* (the wise primate) for our capacity to reason, make moral decisions, and form social groups. These capacities—spiritual, moral, and social—have become key areas of brain research, which studies everything from the exotic effects of hallucinogenic drugs to how brain damage alters morals.

ORIGINS OF RELIGIOUS EXPERIENCE

Hallucinogenic Drugs

Ancient and modern accounts of mystical experiences associated with the use of hallucinogenic drugs are well known. The clinical knowledge that brain seizures are often linked to religious experiences is also long-standing. Against this historical backdrop, recent neuroscience has used functional brain imaging to clarify further that religious and spiritual experiences, like all other human experiences, are grounded in neural processes.

Ancient religious rituals used plants to facilitate ecstatic and mystical states. Mushrooms were used by the Aztecs, peyote cactus by the Huicol of Mexico, and ayahuasca by the natives of northwestern South America. Such uses also extended to water lilies, mandrake, opium poppies, morning glories, and marijuana plants. When these drugs act on particular parts of the brain, researchers believe, they can reveal mechanism that might also be involved in experiences that people describe as religious.

Hallucinogenic substances used in religious ceremonies (with the exception of marijuana) all contain chemicals that fall into one of three categories: tryptamines, phenethylamines, and ergolines. These chemicals affect a complex array of interactive brain systems. At this stage of research, the relationships between the sites and mechanisms of drug action and the subjective (and, in some cases, religious) experiences elicited by the drugs are merely speculative. Nevertheless, a few of the major brain systems stand out in this process.

For example, the three categories of drug all activate the serotonin system of the brain, creating a variety of changes in brain activity. Neurons in a midbrain nucleus (called the raphé) have been found to reduce their firing rate under the influence of these drugs, similar to what occurs during dreaming sleep. The cerebral cortex is also affected by these drugs. Cortical excitability is enhanced by increased release of the excitatory neurotransmitter, glutamate. The thalamus (just below the cortex) also has many serotonin receptors, particularly a small midline area called the reticular nucleus. Drug-related changes in this area alter the way networks in the cerebral cortex give attention to sensory information. It is hypothesized that the effects of hallucinogens on this sensory gating system would create a great deal more sensory noise in cortical information processing.

Another area in the midbrain (the locus coeruleus) is also affected by hallucinogenic drugs. This area is involved in the detection of novel and salient stimuli in the external world. As a hallucinogenic drug changes the processing in this nucleus, a person might take normal everyday stimuli to be extraordinarily significant. Hallucinogens affect yet another area of the midbrain: the ventral tegmental area, which sends dopamine-releasing fibers to the cortical and subcortical structures. The increased dopamine makes events seem biologically significant and activates memory systems.[1]

We are still on very speculative ground here. However, based on what is known about the systems that hallucinogenics act upon and the possible changes that result, some researchers suggest that the drugs

> perturb the key brain structures that inform us about our world, tell us when to pay attention, and interpret what is real. Psychedelics activate ancient brain systems that project to all of the forebrain structures that are involved in memory and feeling; they sensitize systems that tell us when something is novel and when to remember it.[2]

The common subjective experiences elicited by these drugs-related changes in brain systems include

> altered perception of reality and self; intensification of mood; visual and auditory hallucinations, including vivid eidetic imagery and synesthesia; distorted sense of

time and space; enhanced profundity and meaningfulness; and a ubiquitous sense of novelty.[3]

Given the profundity of such experiences, it is natural that subjects will interpret them in various ways. Was it a psychedelic "trip" or an episode of spiritual transcendence? We believe that the interpretation hinges on three things: the individual's experience-based expectations, the setting in which the drugs are taken, and the cognitive/theological network out of which one provides a post-hoc interpretation of the experience.

Temporal Lobe Epilepsy

There is a significant literature in clinical neurology that suggests that, in some cases, individuals with temporal lobe epileptic seizures experience intense religious states as a part of the aura leading up to a seizure. Here, the intense experiences of religious awe, ecstasy, or an ominous presence may be a product of the brain's abnormal electrical activity that brings on the seizures. Although such cases are rare, they happen often enough to suggest something about the physical processes that may be associated with normal religious experiences.

Since the days of belief in a "sacred disease," this phenomenon has received many treatments in literature. At the beginning of this book, we quoted Fyodor Dostoyevsky (who himself had a seizure disorder). He gives a particularly graphic description of this sort of seizure experience told by his character Prince Myshkin in *The Idiot*. A very recent literary treatment can be found in modern novelist Mark Salzman's book, *Lying Awake* (2000). Salzman writes about a nun with religious visions associated with temporal lobe seizures. Patients have also offered their own accounts to the modern-day neurological literature. Here is one that describes the aura experience preceding a seizure:

> Triple halos appeared around the sun. Suddenly the sunlight became intense. I experienced a revelation of

God and of all creation glittering under the sun. The sun became bigger and engulfed me. My mind, my whole being was pervaded by a feeling of delight.[4]

Although such clinical reports are rare, they have led neurologist V. S. Ramachandran to speculate regarding the possible existence of a "God Module" in the brain—that is, "dedicated neural machinery in the temporal lobes concerned with religion."[5] However, we believe UCLA neurologists Jeffery Saver and John Rabin provide a more temperate conclusion in their "limbic marker hypothesis" of religious experiences.

They hypothesize that the limbic (emotional) system of the temporal lobe tags certain encounters as "crucially important, harmonious, and/or joyous, prompting comprehension of these experiences within a religious framework."[6] Whatever the most appropriate statement of the meaning of this phenomenon, it is clear that certain patterns of electrical activity involving the temporal lobes (sometimes occurring during a seizure) can cause intense, personally significant experiences that some persons describe as religious.

Brain Stimulation, Imaging, and Genetics
Abnormal activity of the temporal lobes can be induced artificially in nonepileptic individuals using a noninvasive procedure called Transcranial Magnetic Stimulation. Canadian neuroscientist Michael Persinger reports experiments where electromagnetic stimulation of the right temporal lobe resulted in the person's reporting a "sense of presence." Some subjects take this "presence" to be God, angels, or other supernatural persons. This led Persinger to suggest that all persons who have religious experiences are having microseizures of the right temporal lobe. A similar explanation is given by Persinger for other paranormal experiences, such as reports of encounters with aliens.[7]

It takes a very large leap to go from such preliminary research to a sweeping claim about religious experiences, and some find it completely unwarranted. Still, here is one more suggestion that magnetically induced change in temporal lobes might produce extraordinary experiences. Interestingly, a group of scientists led by Swedish psychologist of religion Pehr Granqvist were unable to replicate Persinger's findings. Instead, they concluded that when religious experiences occurred, these were more determined by situational priming, prior cognitive schemas, and personality dispositions than by temporal lobe stimulation.[8]

Andrew Newberg and his collaborators have also studied brain activity during various religious states. In these studies, they observed changes in regional cerebral blood flow using Single Photon Emission Computed Tomography (SPECT scans). They first studied religious meditation in both Buddhist monks and Catholic nuns. In both groups, the results showed increased activation of both frontal lobes and decreased activity of the right parietal lobe, at the point in time where the meditators reported reaching a state of total absorption and "oneness." Decreased activity of the right parietal lobe was interpreted as the neurological basis of the absence of a sense of self that is sometimes experienced in such meditative states.[9]

As described earlier, the fMRI research of Spezio and colleagues compared brain activity during centering prayer *when* attending to the reading of a narrative passage (chapter 4, Figure 4). Interestingly, these investigators found the opposite results—that is, the right parietal lobe was more active during this form of religious experience.[10] Similarly, Azari and colleagues also found increased right parietal activity during Christian prayer as indicated in PET scans of brain activity.[11] Both of these studies found increased frontal lobe activity, as did Newberg.

Newberg and his colleagues also researched a religious state very different from meditation: the ecstatic religious state involving glossolalia (speaking in tongues). They compared this state to merely singing along with gospel music. Activity in the frontal lobes decreased significantly during glossolalia, consistent with the self-report of loss of intentional control of behavior in this state. This change in the frontal lobes is opposite to that seen during meditation. Decreased activity was also observed in the left temporal pole and left caudate nucleus. In contrast to the reduced right parietal activity seen during meditative states, glossolalia was associated with increased activity in the left superior parietal area.[12]

Thus, these studies suggest both that religious states are associated with identifiable changes in the distribution of brain activity and that different religious states are associated with different patterns of brain activity—in some cases, quite opposite changes in brain activity.

Brain activity, meanwhile, takes place in a biological brain structure that is determined to some degree by the genetic make-up of each person. Thus, it is not unreasonable to suspect that genetic inheritance also affects the religious tendencies of persons. Psychological geneticist (and Episcopal priest) Lindon Eaves has done interesting work suggesting that genes influence our religious characteristics.[13] The evidence comes from comparisons of religious lives of identical and fraternal twins. Identical twins, who share 100 percent of their genetic inheritance, are more alike in their transcendent experiences than are fraternal twins (who share only 50 percent of their genes). Similar outcomes were found for various religious practices such as church attendance. It seems that some aspects of our personal religious tendencies are influenced, at least in some small degree, by our genetic endowment.

The Brain, Religiousness—and Baseball

Whether drug-induced, seizure-related, magnetically stimulated, or born of normal brain processes, our religious states and experiences are clearly intimately tied to our physical brain. What do we make of this relationship?

Ramachandran has made the strongest claim in maintaining that there exists within the temporal lobe a "God module" in the form of a neural area dedicated to religious experiences. In essence, he believes that increased activity in this brain area would be necessary and sufficient for a person to have a religious experience. Thus, if this area becomes abnormally active during a seizure, the person will necessarily have a religious experience and not some other form of experience. This would be the case regardless of the person's prior life experiences, expectancies, habitual ways of interpreting his or her life experiences, and the environmental context in which the seizure occurs. Thus, religious experiences are, in the view of Ramachandran, a unique and intrinsic class of experiences served by a unique brain structure.

A different interpretation of the same clinical data was offered by Saver and Rabin. They argue that certain temporal lobe seizures activate a brain system that evokes feelings of deep significance, harmoniousness, joy, etc. Whether the experience is described in religious terms is a product of the prior experiences and interpretive networks of the person having the seizure. This explains why some persons have temporal lobe seizures that have similar *experiential qualities* but are not described or experienced by the person as religious.

This interpretation is consistent with the theory of religious experiences offered by the early twentieth-century American psychologist William James in his 1902 study *The Varieties of Religious Experience*. According to James, differences in the religious (or non-religious) interpretations given by persons to mundane or unusual experiences are related to culturally inherited "over-beliefs." Religious meaning is not intrinsic to the experience but applied by the interpretive network of the experiencer. In the physical brain, therefore, we don't need to hypothesize a so-called God module. More likely, we are seeing something like this: a temporal lobe seizure activates a complex process in a local, general-purpose neural network, and this network then weaves those abnormal signals into the brain's broader pattern of prior beliefs and understandings.

In this light, Persinger's work with magnetic stimulation also fails to establish that a specific part of the brain is dedicated to religious experiences. Persinger's key finding is that subjects experience a sense of the presence of another person. Again, this is more likely to be the activity of a general-purpose brain network that is dedicated to our feeling that the presence of a person is more significant than the presence of a chair or dog. The Persinger experiments could be explained this way: under the magnetic stimulation, subjects must reconcile the activation of their presence-detecting neural network with the fact that they have no sensory data that a physical person is actually present. If the subjects have a worldview that includes spiritual beings (or aliens), he or she might interpret the brain signals as the presence of God, an angel, a ghost, or an alien. As James would tell us, a particular form of over-belief is necessary for any brain experience to be given a religious interpretation.

Newberg's studies of meditation prompted him to conclude at first that the brain is wired for religious experiences. As he titled his 2001 book, that is why "God won't go away." However, his studies of glossolalia undermined the idea that one particular brain module or wiring system produces religious experiences. Different forms of religious experience, it seems, arise from different parts of the brain. In sum, there is no single brain area where greater or lesser activity is necessary and sufficient to produce what people would take to be a religious experience. These changes in brain activity, as found in imaging studies, are not unique to a religious experience. However, the mind may certainly interpret the activity in these more general neural systems as a kind of religious state, colored by the religious context of the experience and the personal history of the individual.

This leads us to an important conclusion. In our view, religion cannot be reduced to a *primary* form of cognitive activity, such as can be done for language (which has identifiable neural systems and structures). Rather, "religion" is more like "baseball"—a cultural and social phenomenon that includes a variety of individual and group experiences, events, and activities. Baseball encompasses the group participation of players and spectators. Players use their motor skills. Fans get caught up in baseball as a topic of continual interest, conversation, and attendance. Baseball involves moments of intense emotion (not unlike a moment of religious ecstasy). It also has ritual-like activity (think of pregame and between-inning warmup for players, the seventh-inning stretch, and singing the national anthem). Baseball involves complex layers of interpersonal and social organization and thus is a better model for religion than a cognitive process like language.

With baseball as a conceptual model for religion, the neurological study of religion changes its approach. First, we would not expect to find a specific neurology of baseball—that is, no unique neurological systems that would contribute specifically to baseball and not to other forms of life. Baseball is neither sufficiently unitary as an experience nor sufficiently embodied in biology to study at the level of neurology. Second, we would not expect to find a neurological disorder specific to baseball, although such a disorder in a person might alter the participation and appreciation of the sport. Third, it would be somewhat far-fetched to imagine the evolution of the specific capacity for baseball or to argue for the survival advantages of baseball to individuals or social groups or to argue that the specific capacity for baseball is "hard wired." Rather, baseball is a complex social phenomenon. The reality of baseball "emerges" as it piggy-backs its activities and experiences—cognitively, neurologically, and evolutionarily—onto a large number of more general cognitive capacities and skills.[14]

This leads to the further question as to whether religion is essentially individual or corporate. Does it arise only within individual persons, or is it generated between persons (or persons and social contexts)? If religion is primarily interpersonal, social, and cultural, then it cannot be found at the level of neurology, except in the human being's more general cognitive and psychosocial functions—those that are used in interpersonal and social interactions. The neural events involved in religious experiences and behaviors overlap with too many other nonreligious and subjective experiences. If religion is primarily social, there cannot be a neurology of specific religious behaviors or experiences. There could only be a neurology that would look at brain systems that guide individuals as social beings, and then look specifically in the context of religion, as W. S. Brown argues. This approach, of course, makes the reality of a "religion nucleus" or a "God module" very unlikely and a "neuroscience of religion" or "neurotheology" very implausible.

MORAL DECISION MAKING

What about morality? Is it a unique spiritual feature of human nature, or is it a quality that overlaps with other operations of the brain and body? For those who hold the view of body–soul dualism, the moral life of the person is presumed to happen primarily in the soul, not the body. A nondualist view presumes the brain/body is making moral decisions, although we are not entirely clear on how brain systems do this. In either case, people's moral behaviors often are guided by their worldviews and religious perspectives, and so we typically say that religion and morality go hand-in-hand.

Theories of moral behavior in both philosophy and in moral psychology generally can be classified either as (1) those that emphasize the processes (largely conscious) involved in making rational choices or (2) those that emphasize virtue and character. The former theories view moral decision making as a cognitive process similar to calculation of interests, weighing potential outcomes or deciding what might be good for oneself and for others. The latter theories emphasize the fact that real-time moral behavior does not seem to involve such calculations, and the press-of-events usually means one responds automatically, without really thinking about it. In such cases, morality would be a matter of habitual responses that are often summarized as constituting a person's character, virtuous or otherwise.

From a nondualist point of view, both of these theoretical

approaches—morality as "process" versus morality as "virtue"—presume that various brain systems are at work in regulating behavior. Here are some examples of our attempts to understand those brain systems.

The Frontal Lobes

The story of Phineas Gage, first mentioned in chapter 5, is perhaps the most famous single case in all of neurology when it comes to the study of the brain and morality. The brain injury suffered by Gage and its outcome illustrates the impact on moral capacity of damage to the frontal lobe of the brain, particularly to the lower-middle portion of the frontal lobe known as the orbital frontal cortex. This case also illustrates the importance of the brain's unconscious, automatic emotional guidance of behavior—the part of our moral lives that we refer to as character or virtue.

Gage received major damage to his frontal lobes when an iron bar that he was using to tamp an explosive charge was blown up through his eye-socket and out the top of his head. While Gage never lost consciousness and seemed to have recovered physically within days, he was never the same person. Prior to the accident, he was a person of admirable character—a capable and efficient worker, excellent manager, responsible family man, and upstanding citizen. While he maintained his general intelligence after the accident, damage to his frontal cortex resulted in an interpersonal style best described as unreliable and capricious, socially inappropriate, and amoral.

Study of other patients with this form of brain damage shows that they typically have difficulty regulating their behavior in order to abide by norms of socially acceptable or moral behavior. Such individuals may, capriciously and without malicious intent, violate social conventions, laws, ethical standards, or the rules of courtesy, civility, and regard for the benefit of others.

Neurologist Antonio Damasio has done a great deal of study of individuals with injury to the orbital frontal cortex of the brain.

Out of this research, he developed the theory of somatic markers as an explanation of what goes wrong in this sort of brain injury, as explained in his work *Descartes' Error: Emotion, Reason, and the Human Brain* (1994). According to this theory, our life experiences help our minds develop automatic responses to events—what we shall call anticipatory-evaluative-affective responses. These are coupled to our knowledge of the world. At moments when our consciousness lacks the relevant knowledge for a decision, we are guided by subtle emotions and intuitions. These might include feeling suspicions toward a person or feeling that a certain behavior might not be the right thing to do. In many circumstances, these autonomic responses guide our behavior.

Damasio believes that damage to the orbital frontal cortex decouples conscious decision making from our more autonomic emotional response systems. Usually, when we consider an action, we can recall (unconsciously) whether it had negative consequences in a previous experience. This also comes to us automatically as a negative emotional signal. Brain damage stops this signal—our evaluative emotional response. Without this, behavior loses its anchor in previous experiences and becomes capricious. The implication of Damasio's theory is that our emotions deliver many of our most complex and rational judgments about the world, guiding us in our moment-to-moment decision making. Without knowing why, we often just feel that this or that is the right thing to do in this situation.

Brain Activity and Moral Decisions

Neuroscience is also mapping brain areas involved in different forms of interpersonal, economic, and moral decision making. This type of research uses functional magnetic resonance imaging (fMRI) to scan a subject's brain as he or she engages in decision-making tasks. For example, studies have demonstrated that the brain's limbic (emotional) area is quite active even when a subject is making a "cold" calculation, such as the likelihood of financial gains and losses. In fact, the limbic involvement is particularly intense when the financial decision involves interpersonal variables such as trust.

Using similar fMRI techniques, Harvard psychologist Joshua Greene and his collaborators have studied moral decision making. Their first studies observed how activity in certain brain areas increased as subjects were presented with more difficult moral dilemmas. The activity especially increased on the lateral frontal lobes and limbic cortex. A follow-up study presented still harder moral dilemmas: would the subjects directly, or indirectly, harm one person in order to save the lives of many others? When they imagined these two kinds of choices, the brain showed two different patterns of activity. Decisions about whether to inflict harm directly on someone, for example, activated brain areas more involved in modulating social action and representations of the self.[15]

These kinds of studies are showing us that moral regulation of behavior is an embodied process. Different forms of moral decision making involve different patterns of brain activity. Nevertheless, as we will discuss later, this does not imply a deterministic process controlling our human choices, as if they are the inevitable outcome of lower-level neurobiological processes. The human nervous system is a highly complex and dynamic system that allows persons (as whole beings) to generate choices that are real and have a form of freedom.

Social Neuroscience

Damasio's somatic marker theory is part of a wider field of research called "social neuroscience," because it deals with interpersonal relations. The somatic marker theory, for example, suggests that moral behavior arises both from feelings toward others (for example, empathy or compassion) and from feelings about the nature of a situation (unfairness or social inclusion/exclusion). Here are some more examples of what clinical phenomena and research are telling us about the neurological basis of human relationships.

Perceptions of Relatedness

Capgras syndrome is a disorder of the experience of familiarity when encountering close friends and family. In these rare cases, damage to parts of the temporal lobe can result in a disorder characterized by the individual's conviction that close friends or family members are not really themselves but are "doubles" and impostors. A family member, when encountered, may be visually recognized in such a way as to say, "That person looks like my wife." However, it is believed that, because of the damage to the temporal lobes, the person with Capgras syndrome does not experience the accompanying feeling of familiarity and deep personal regard typically associated with the visual perception of a loved one. Therefore, the patient presumes that the family member or friend in question must be an impostor —"not really my wife." Capgras syndrome demonstrates that these feelings of familiarity (and love) can be dissociated from the visual recognition of the identity of the person by a dysfunction of the temporal lobes of the brain.[16]

Theory of Mind Revisited

Critical to personal relatedness is the capacity to infer accurately and understand the mental states of other persons. In psychology, this ability is often referred to as a "theory of mind," as we discussed in the previous chapter. This ability involves knowing and understanding what the other person knows, intends, feels, and is likely to do. Much of the current interest in the concept of a theory of mind has come about due to the speculation that individuals with autism and Asperger's syndrome have a specific deficiency in this capacity. Both of these disorders are characterized by a deficit in comprehending and responding to the social and emotional nature of situations.[17]

The ability to understand the intentions and social emotions of other people by their actions also seems to be lost in autism. Neuropsychologists Uta Frith and Fulvia Castelli, working in London, have studied this by comparing how individuals with and without autism infer intentions and emotions from the movements of geometric figures in simple animations. The research confirmed this deficit in autistic individuals. The studies also showed that when subjects do infer "interpersonal" intentionality in impersonal actions, such as triangles interacting on a computer screen, the areas of brain activity are the medial frontal cortex and the superior temporal lobe.[18]

Experiences of Unfairness

The concept of fairness is an important and very high-level aspect of human interpersonal interactions and moral considerations. Psychologist Alan Sanfey and his colleagues have conducted functional brain scans on participants in the so-called "ultimatum game," in which two people split a sum of money. One player proposes a division of the money and the other person (whose brain is being scanned) can accept or reject the offer. The experience of being given what is perceived to be an unfair division of the money shows up as a particular pattern of brain activity (which include the right frontal cortex and areas in the limbic cortex that process emotion).[19] Further fMRI studies have used economic games to observe the development of trust between participants. They have shown that a player's intention to trust (on the next round of the game) can be predicted by both the timing and magnitude of activity in a brain area called the dorsal striatum, underlying the cerebral cortex.[20]

Another social experience that is related to fairness is the experience of being socially included or excluded from a group of other persons. Brain scans of individuals who are being included in or excluded from a virtual-reality game show that exclusion is accompanied by activation in the cingulate cortex and the right frontal cortex.[21]

Empathy

Empathy is an interpersonal emotion that regulates our engagement in certain forms of moral behavior. Recent fMRI research by neuroscientist Tania Singer found that subjects empathizing with the pain of a friend or spouse show active brain patterns in the same areas that light up when the subjects themselves experience pain.[22] Specifically, empathy-related activation occurs within the limbic (emotional) cortex associated with the emotional consequences of pain, but not with that part of the brain that processes the bodily sensation of actual physical pain. Thus, empathy represents an attunement of one's own emotional systems with the perceived emotional experiences of the other person.

As we have suggested, these physical correlations of brain and body with religious experiences, moral decisions, and deep interpersonal relatedness conflict with the sentiments held by many that our "soul," a nonmaterial thing, is the source of such experiences. Nevertheless, the role of brain function, brain damage, brain stimulation, and even genetics is hard to deny in many of these intuitions and behaviors.

Modern theologians have taken note of this obvious clash of viewpoints. German theologian Wolfhart Pannenberg, for example, has pointedly asked, "When the life of the soul is conditioned in every detail by bodily organs and processes, how can it be detached from the body and survive it?"[23] He believes that modern believers must reconsider dualism in the face of the mounting evidence: the many studies of neurological damage and disease and the many laboratory experiments on brain functions linked to our most human behaviors. This abandonment of dualistic "soul" can be hard medicine. But, as we will show later, there is an alternative—there is a scientifically informed way to preserve belief in personhood and moral agency and the truth of religious experience.

CHAPTER 8
Science, Religion, and Human Nature

WHAT ARE THE implications of new scientific research for a theological understanding of human nature? Although the evidence of the embodied mind has grown, it continues to be critically evaluated, and there is still no knockdown, indisputable argument, no conclusive proof that body/soul or mind/brain dualism are wrong or that a nuanced view of mind/brain interdependence is right. While there is a general consensus among neuroscientists in favor of the physical embodiment of mind, as we saw earlier, distinguished scientists can be lined up on both sides of the argument.

Nevertheless, given accumulating evidence of embodiment, we must explore the implications that a "physicalist" understanding of persons has for theological views of human nature. Embodiment raises the question of whether we are free to think and act as we wish. In other words, are our thoughts and behaviors "nothing but the meaningless motion of molecules," a notion lamented by the Christian physicist and psychologist Donald MacKay?[1] Both religious persons and nonreligious humanists agree that the idea of moral responsibility and culpability rests heavily upon the assumption that we are agents who choose our own actions. Therefore, we must examine carefully how best to think about human agency and free will.

This idea of human freedom has long underwritten the case that humans are distinctive from other animals. As the Christian tradition asserts, human are made "in the image of God." Historically, one of the most enduring views is that this *imago dei* in humans is the capacity to use reason. Another historical view is that humans are unique by their capacity for moral agency. As we noted earlier, evolutionary psychology has questioned whether reason is really exclusive to the human species. It has also begun to probe the question of whether other creatures behave in ways that might be called "moral" or, at least, altruistic.

NEUROSCIENCE ON HUMAN NATURE

While body/soul dualism is the most prevalent view of human nature within historical Christianity, this view comes less from biblical sources than from a line of philosophical theories that can be traced from Plato to Saint Augustine to René Descartes. Descartes is most responsible for solidifying this dualist position into a strong categorical body/mind (or body/soul) distinction.

Despite his dualism, Descartes was mostly a physicalist. He did not believe that the body was inhabited by many souls, or nonmaterial forces, that controlled bodily functions, as was commonly believed in his time. Rather, he believed that bodily functions were best understood as a physical "machine." He presumed that the functioning of animals did not transcend these mechanisms. The problem for Descartes was figuring out how such a biological mechanism could result in human reason. He solved this problem by retaining one soul—the rational mind. Thus, humans were considered to be different from animals in having a rational soul that was immaterial and interacted with the physical body through the pineal gland.

It is reasonable to speculate that Descartes would probably have seen rationality as embodied in brain function if he had had the modern data of neuroscience. He would have been able to see (1) mind/brain links, (2) the overlap of some cognitive capacity between humans and other primates, and (3) the neural embodiment of religious experiences and moral decision making. But it was probably impossible for Descartes to imagine such a unitary (physicalist) view of human nature because this sophisticated knowledge was not yet available.

Now that we have that information, the abandonment of the Cartesian viewpoint is only natural. A variety of modern theories of human nature has attempted to do this by formulating alternatives to the older Cartesian dualism. The most materialist, and thus radical, is an approach called *eliminative materialism*. This view asserts that all causes of human behavior are entirely reducible to physics, the electrical and chemical actions underlying neurology. This is an extremely *reductionist* view. Its scientific proponents dismiss the mental aspects of belief and decision as having any important role in explaining human behavior. A very similar view goes by the term *epiphenomenalism*, which proposes that conscious mental life, and the experience of making decisions and doing things for reasons, is merely an inconsequential by-product of what the microstructures of the brain are doing.

We can sense how reductionist this epiphenomenalist view can be when we consider it is opposed by many leading researchers, including three Nobel laureates who have argued for the primacy of consciousness behavior (a top-down processes, versus the bottom-up process of neurons alone). As neurophysiologist Sir John Eccles once wrote, "Let us be clear that for each of us the primary reality is consciousness—everything else is derivative and has a second order quality."[2] Neurobiologist Gerald Edelman makes the case that in biology, "the evolutionary assumption implies that consciousness is *efficacious*—that it is *not* an epiphenomenon."[3] And neuropsychologist Roger Sperry wrote, "The new model [in neuroscience] adds a downward to the traditional upward microdeterminism and is claimed to give science a conceptual foundation that is more adequate, valid and comprehensive."[4] All these views are endorsed by the Oxford mathematician Sir Roger Penrose, who wrote that "consciousness is the phenomenon whereby the universe's very existence is made known."[5]

Given this debate between top-down and bottom-up advocates,

where does the physicalist view of human nature stand? Although the physicalist stance aims for a unitary and embodied understanding of the mind, it does not necessarily presume that mental life must be reduced only to chemistry and physics. Instead, it supports a range of theories that operate under the heading of *nonreductive physicalism*. In this view, while humans are taken to be entirely physical, the brain is seen as complex enough to support the emergence of mental properties and experiences that have a real influence on behavior.[6] A similar view, but with a different emphasis, is *dual-aspect monism*. The term *monism* means, in this context, essentially the same thing as *physicalism*. But the modifier *dual-aspect* emphasizes the fact that an adequate description of human nature must entail at least two levels (or aspects)—a physical description provided by neuroscience and a mental description as represented in our subjective experiences and studied by psychology. Finally, there is a view called *emergent dualism*. Here, the physical reality is taken as first and primary but then from it emerges a completely new entity—a mind or soul. This might seem like it circles back to the dualism of Descartes, but it is actually different: it gives the physical side precedence.

REDUCTIONISM, DETERMINISM, AND EMERGENCE

In order to escape eliminative materialism without resorting to dualism (as Descartes had done) one needs to deal with two issues—reductionism and determinism. Reductionism is the idea that all higher-level causes (for example, the cause of a specific human behavior) can be reduced to nothing more than the outcome of the laws operating at lower levels (namely, the laws governing the neurochemistry of neurons). This form of reductionism has been brought to biology from physics.

According to this view, all the original causes of behavior are found at the level of atomic and subatomic matter. That explanation is taken as sufficient. Accordingly, the organism as a whole is seen as playing no role in organizing, directing, or influencing its own behavior. Since all the physical forces are atomic and subatomic and since the physical world is a causally closed system (as the story goes), the ideas of human agency and moral behavior are deemed incoherent. Faced with such stark reductionism, the only way to explain moral agency and personal responsibility is to resort to Descartes' option—add a nonmaterial part (a mind or soul) that is not subject to a reductive view of physical processes.

Fortunately, we don't have to become Cartesians all over again. There are, in fact, reasons to believe that systems, even though made up of elements obeying the laws of physics, can embody forms of causation that transcend the determinism of these atomic and chemical laws. We can understand and defend this idea of a larger causal system by the use of two concepts: *emergence* and its partner, *top-down causation*. Together, they sketch out how mental processes and moral agency can be the real causes of behavior and yet, at the same time, be embodied in a biological system.

Emergence[7]

The concept of emergence refers to the possibility that complex entities (like organisms) can have properties that do not exist within the elements (such as molecules) that make up the complex entity. Thus, even an amoeba, as a complex organization of molecules, has properties that do not exist in the molecules themselves. The activity of the amoeba is governed by the current state of the organization of these molecules, not the properties of the molecules themselves. Hence, the activity of the amoeba is an emergent property.

Another term for emergence is *dynamical systems theory*. It attempts to explain how new causal properties (whether the behavior of amoebas or humans) can emerge in complex systems that are characterized by a high level of nonlinear interactions between their elements. A perfect example is the human cerebral cortex.

Its millions of neurons and massive number of interconnections are ideally suited for a dynamical system. From the countless separate pieces of human neurobiology, the cerebral cortex produces the high-level (and nonreductive) cognitive properties of a whole person.

The ant colony is another analogy for how complex dynamical systems produce new, whole-system properties. Of course, an ant colony cannot support the emergence of something like human cognition. But that is not only because ants are "mindless"; it's because the complexity of ant social interactions are vastly less complex than that of neurons in the brain! Still, we can imagine individual ants as analogous to individual neurons. That makes the colony something like a brain, where the emergent properties exceed the ability of individual ants.

Ant colonies (as colonies) show various forms of "intelligent" behavior. They manage to locate the trash pile and the cemetery at points where they are closest to each other and also at points where both are closest to the ant colony itself. Hence, the ants have solved a spatial mathematical problem. Colonies also solve the problem of the shortest distance to a source of food. They prioritize food sources. But who is doing the solving? The solution is beyond the capacity of individual ants. Most interestingly, colonies modify their behavior over time. Colonies as a whole go through stages, progressively changing their colony-level behavior. Young colonies are more persistent and aggressive, but also more fickle, than older ones.

Each individual ant, however, operates by a set of simple rules of responding to information from the social and physical environment. A great deal of work has gone into describing these rules. The question is whether the rules governing individual ant behavior are sufficient to explain all of the colony behavior or whether there are properties of colony behavior that are emergent and cannot be reduced to the rules governing individuals ants. Dynamical systems theory gives us a way to understand how both complex whole-ant-colony behavior and higher-order human cognition can emerge from the interactions of less complex elements (ants or neurons).

When environmental change pushes complex dynamical systems (such as ant colonies or human brains) away from equilibrium, they self-organize (and progressively reorganize) into new interactive patterns to deal with the new environment. These new patterns form as the interactive elements (individual ants or neurons) constrain each other's activity. Individual elements start working in a coordinated manner, and the probability of each element's doing one thing or another is altered by its interactions with all of the other elements. Hence, an *aggregate* of individual elements (ants or neurons) becomes a new dynamical *system* (a colony with particular colony-wise properties or a brain with cognitive properties). Once this system is organized, its lower-level properties (rules of individual ant behavior or of neuron firing) interact bottom-up with the top-down relational constraints. This bottom-top interaction creates higher-level patterns (colony coordination or whole-brain functioning) without any change in the physical laws at microlevels (within individual ants or neurons).

By adapting to a changing environment, these dynamic systems embody what we can call *meaning*. That is, the state of organization of the system carries forward a "memory" of previous interactions with its environment embodied in its current organization. On the basis of previous organizations and reorganizations in response, the system is more adequately prepared to deal with similar situations in the future.

These constant reorganizations of the system do more than just adapt to a changing environment: they create increasingly more complex forms of organization. Multiple smaller systems can be reorganized into a larger system. The process creates a nested hierarchy of more and more complex emergent functional systems. Paradoxically, the *constraints* that lower-level elements (ants) put on each other help produce *greater freedom* at the higher level of the system as a whole (colony). The system develops a substantially greater number of possible interactions with its environment than it had in each preceding step of self-reorganization.

The most interesting property of complex, nonlinear, dynamical systems is that they manifest novelty. The behavior of the entire system, even given a stable environment, is not entirely predictable. Even in small-scale mathematical models of dynamical systems, no two runs of the same system model ever come out exactly the same. Considering all these features of dynamical systems, they become perfect models for our understanding of the human brain. We can imagine how the physical brain produces truly causal emergent properties that cannot be explained by the lower operation of physics, chemistry, and neurons.

Top-down Causation

As we've already appreciated, higher-level emergent properties have a *top-down influence* on constituent parts of a system—our second important concept in understanding the dynamic brain. As a system self-organizes under environmental change, it puts new constrains, as if top-down controls, on the future states of its individual parts. In the case of ants, the characteristics of the entire colony have top-down influences on the behavior of the individuals. With respect to human brain systems, microlevel processes (the physics and chemistry of neurons) become caught up in, and influenced by, the larger dynamic patterns that constitute the ebb and flow of activity of the brain as a whole.

In summary, we can draw two conclusions about brain function: (1) the emergent phenomena of mental activity—thinking, deciding, consciousness, memory, language, representation, belief—operate as shifting patterns in a dynamical neural system and (2) such patterns create top-down influences on the lower-level neurophysiological phenomena that support the mental activities themselves. When viewed this way, future discussions of the human brain will need an entirely new language to describe its "mentalist" operations as a whole, especially as they emerge from the exceedingly complex cerebral cortex. The brain realizes the optimal physical conditions for the emergence of a complex dynamic system in the following ways:

1. a high degree of complexity in the form of a very large number of elements (neurons)
2. maximal interconnectivity of elements (a very large number of branches of dendrites and axons, and even larger numbers of synapses per neuron)
3. a great deal of two-way interaction between elements (called recurrent connectivity)
4. nonlinear interactions that serve to amplify small perturbations or small differences in initial conditions.

The brain has one more fascinating feature. As a dynamic system, its structure modifies itself at the level of cellular interactions, which are the synapses. This moment-by-moment interaction can change entire patterns in the brain system long into the future. The brain takes on what researchers call its plasticity, or ability to reorganize and grow in mental capacity.

We have already introduced in chapter 4 the "dynamic core theory" of consciousness proposed by Gerald Edleman and Giulio Tononi. Their model is another example of the brain's having emergent properties. They argue that consciousness (and its content) is a temporary and dynamically changing pattern of functional interconnectedness among widespread cortical areas. This dynamic core is a complex, widespread, and highly differentiated neural state that, from moment to moment, includes different subsets of neurons or neural groups. These specific neural groupings, and the interactions among the groupings, embody the form and content of consciousness at any particular moment.

Edelman and Tononi also argue that dynamic cores (and thus consciousness) are characteristic of the mental life of all animals when the cerebral cortex has sufficiently rich interconnections. As they express it, consciousness becomes possible by a

> transcendent leap from simple nervous systems, in which signals are exchanged in a relatively insulated manner within separate neural subsystems, to complex nervous systems based on reentrant dynamics, in which an enormous number of signals are rapidly integrated within a single neural process constituting the dynamic core. Such integration leads to the construction of a scene relating signals from many different modalities with memory based on an entire evolutionary history and an individual's experience—it is a remembered present. This scene integrates and generates an extraordinary amount of information within less than a second.[8]

Thus, what Edelman and Tononi are describing as the basis of consciousness is a dynamically self-organizing complex system within the cerebral cortex, very much like what is described as properties of complex, nonlinear dynamical systems.

Human Uniqueness?

As we have tried to make clear, the atoms, molecules, and cells that make up the body are not enough to explain all animal and human behaviors. These behaviors arise from distinctive new properties that emerge from a neural and cognitive complexity that develops in the context of complex social and cultural environments. The same should hold true for the origin of religious experience. The research seems to show that, with respect to base-level cognitive properties, there is very little that makes humans unique among animals, although humans have obvious enhancements of these mental capacities.

However, human uniqueness does arise at some point: we believe that humans *become* unique by the interaction between these enhanced mental capacities and the complexity and uniqueness of human society and culture. Some of our best scientists are probing how this complexity of mind and environment works. In 2007, the paleoanthropologist Alison Brooks argued that "social intelligence" requires six different faculties. These can be listed as: abstract thought; the ability to cooperate in forward planning; problem solving through behavioral, economic, and technological innovation; "imagined communities"; symbolic thinking; and a "theory of mind" (a key feature of which is the ability to understand that other individuals may have ideas and desires different from one's own). Hence "social intelligence" emerges from the integrative use of a suite of more base-level cognitive capacities. According to Brooks, each of these capacities has a long phylogenetic history of development. Humanness appeared as gradual process, she says, so "the more we know, the harder it is to draw a line between human and nonhuman or pre-human."[9]

Recent evidence from paleoanthropology underlines this view. For example, the best current understanding of physical, behavioral, and cultural indicators of humanness shows that they appeared thousands of years before humans were present in the Middle East. Brooks argues that "the capabilities for living in 'our heads' [as self-consciousness] were present before 130,000 years ago and developed in a step-wise fashion, possibly in a feedback relationship with our morphology." The capabilities she includes as having already appeared in at least a primitive form are "some of the most human qualities: creativity, empathy, reverence, spirituality, aesthetic appreciation, abstract thought, and problem-solving (rationality). [These] were already evident soon after the emergence of our species."[10] The meaning of *reverence* and *spirituality* may be debated but are relevant in any discussion of the emergence of the *imago dei*.

Based on this view of human and animal nature, how should religious concepts of human uniqueness be understood—or should they be entirely abandoned? In June of 2007, a lead article in the science journal *Nature* proclaimed, "With all deference to the sensibilities of religious people, the idea that man was created in the image of God can surely be put aside."[11] Such headline-grabbing claims are not unfamiliar today in discussions about human nature. The *Nature* article went on to say, "Scientific theories of human nature may be discomforting or unsatisfying, but they are not illegitimate." The first quote is, as we shall see in a moment, not a scientific statement. The second is merely a claim about the current state of scientific theories of human nature that applies as much to the views (and potential discomfort) of a humanist as to those of a religious person.

Given the remarkable successes already achieved in neuroscience, neuropsychology, and evolutionary psychology, it is easy to assume that the scientific approach is the only way of gaining reliable knowledge about ourselves. However, to do so would be to ignore a lively and ongoing debate within science itself about how best to balance the benefits of a reductionist approach to the phenomena we study with the contributions made by less reductionist disciplines such as social science. It seems clear from the view of social science that human behavior cannot simply be reduced to the explanations of biological science nor can biological science be reduced to physical science.

It is a perfectly normal thing for any biologist to refer to the "nature" of particular groups of organisms as they occur in the evolutionary phyla. For example, evolutionary psychologist Andrew Whiten wrote:

> Establishing the "nature" of any species has traditionally been an essentially descriptive exercise aiming to delineate ever more clearly what it is to be a member of that species. . . . Since Darwin, however, we can think of the nature of a species in additional ways; from an

evolutionary perspective, we can ask (for example) what differentiates the nature of a species such as our own from its closest living relatives, and how the difference arose from common origins.[12]

References to species differences would appear on a scale that would include, for example, entomology, rodentology, ornithology, and primatology. Whiten took this approach in his study of what he called a "deep social mind" in humankind: "At a descriptive level, the claim is that human beings are not merely the cleverest species, but also the most social, in the depth of their cognitive interpenetration."[13] Drawing attention to such features is important in the task of classifying organisms. A group of leading scholars, including Whiten, not known for their religious affiliations, have recently suggested features that are uniquely human. The 2008 book *What Makes Us Human?* presents several candidates for which factor is most significant in making us human. The foreword by the distinguished geneticist Walter Bodmer tells us:

> In the various articles you will find suggestions that include the "spirit of man," referring particularly to religion, speech and not just language, imitation and "mimetics," cooking, high levels of cognitive ability, causal belief, that humans are symbolic creatures, innate curiosity and the desire to know, mental time travel, and the ability to read other's minds. These all have cognitive ability as a common thread and, deriving from this, high-level development of language and cultural transmission.[14]

The strength of the evidence offered in support of each of these proposals varies considerably, and it is evident that within the scientific domain we are only at the beginning of the search for answers to the question of what makes us human.

In the religious domain, it is natural and perfectly proper to ask whether there is anything that distinguishes humans from other animals in addition to any distinct physical or cognitive characteristics. This is to ask questions within the domain of religious anthropology, which uses different nonscientific categories. Compared to the scientific list of human characteristics above, a list relevant to Christian theology, for example, would have to add such topics as soteriology, pneumatology, ecclesiology, and Christian anthropology. Religious anthropology is different from scientific or secular anthropology. It involves wider realms of discourse and a different way of seeking to know truth.

A CHANGING STORY: THE "IMAGE OF GOD"

Christian anthropology has traditionally asked what it means to say that humans are made "in the image of God." Over the past two millennia, various thinkers have given different answers, each focusing on a specific quality that seems to makes humans unique, and thus defining the essential meaning of "the image of God."

A Capacity to Reason

One of the most persistent claims to distinctiveness has been our ability to reason. A Roman Catholic catechism avers: "God . . . can be known . . . by the natural light of reason. . . . Man has this capacity because he is created 'in the image of God.'"[15] This notion reflects, in part, the influence of Descartes, who believed that "the human mind, by virtue of its rationality, provides evidence both of a kind of image of God and at the same time a criterion of radical discontinuity from the rest of creation. The animals are merely machines."[16]

Unfortunately for this view, we now know that animals show behaviors that, if we saw them in children, we would say demonstrated simple forms of reasoning and problem-solving—the basis of rationality. Language is a capacity associated with reason that was once thought to be uniquely human. Much recent research has shown clearly that chimpanzees can master language at the level of a two- to three-year-old child, as we have previously mentioned. Investigators have even reported evidence of a rudimentary capacity to use syntax in nonhuman primates.[17] While this is not developed language, it does mean that another apparent Rubicon previously separating us from the rest of the animal kingdom has been crossed.

In addition, there is evidence that animals have at least a rudimentary form of a "theory of mind," the ability to represent themselves in their own mental processes. This ability is inferred from "mirror self-recognition." Such self-recognition is rare in animals, but it has been demonstrated in human children, great apes, dolphins, and elephants. Frans de Waal and his colleagues suggest that such mirror self-recognition "indexes an increased self-other distinction that also underlies the social complexity and altruistic tendencies among these large-brained animals."[18] Bonobos (pygmy chimps) seem to be capable of "thinking about thinking."[19] As described earlier, the research literature is full of results suggesting at least echoes in higher primates of the human-like capacities once thought to be uniquely human.

A Distinctive Role and Relationship

Earlier interpretations about substantive "reason" being unique to humans are being replaced by functional interpretations. One reason for this is that substantive views appear to be too static and too dependent upon a belief in a thinking "substance" called the mind that is distinct and separate from the body. In contrast, however, the Old Testament scholar Gerhard Von Rad has argued that the *imago dei* is found not in what we are, but in what we are called to do. This is the functionalist view of the *imago dei*. It presents humans as having divine status by exercising control and stewardship in the creation.[20]

For others, this human role in nature is not enough to define the *imago dei*. They emphasize instead that humanness is a capacity for

personal relatedness—or, as Whiten puts it, a "deep social mind."
One author of this book (Warren Brown) has taken this position,
arguing that unique forms of human personal relatedness emerge
from the interplay of a suite of enhanced (but not unique) cognitive capacities—such as complex language, mentalizing ("thinking
about thinking"), episodic memory, conscious top-down agency,
future orientation, and emotional modulation of cognition.[21]

Another major theme proposed by those championing the relational aspects of the *imago dei* is the capacity for relationship with
God. For theologian Karl Barth, it is not just a capacity for relationships that is crucial, but it is relationships themselves—that is, a
relationship with God and relationships with each other. In a similar manner, Gerrit Berkouwer argues that the Bible emphasizes the
whole human being as the image of God. Human uniqueness is
grounded in relational action rather than a substantive property:
our love of others makes us concretely in the image of God. Of
course, the capacity for interpersonal relationships is not some
free-floating, nonmaterial capacity or entity. According to social
neuroscience and evolutionary psychology, this capacity is firmly
embodied in ways that we are beginning to understand.

For Old Testament scholar Claus Westermann, "relationship to
God is not something which is added to human existence; humans
are created in such a way that their very existence is intended to be
their relationship to God"; in the Genesis account, only "the man"
is addressed directly by God (Gen. 1:28).[22] Westermann has also
noted,

> the meaning is indisputable. Man in his entirety ... is to
> be designated as a creature in God's image.... [It] serves
> to underline the uniqueness of man's creation. The cre-
> ation of man is something far different from the creation
> of the rest of the world. One can almost say that this rup-
> tures the framework of the course of creation in which all
> the other works of creation are included.[23]

Two of today's most distinguished Christian theologians, Wolfhart Pannenberg and Jurgen Moltmann, add a transcendent and eschatological dimension to the relationship idea. A key word for Pannenberg is *exocentricity*, emphasizing that we are constantly reaching beyond our experiences of the present world in a search for fulfillment and meaning. Moltmann, in turn, believes that there is a fundamental self-transcendence that defines humankind and will ultimately find its proper identity only in Jesus Christ, who fulfills the image of God in its entirety.

A Capacity for Moral Agency

Another interpretation of what makes us in the image of God was accentuated in the eighteenth century by North America's first great theologian, Jonathan Edwards. He emphasized that the capacity for moral behavior and moral agency was a key feature of what it meant to be made in the image of God. He wrote, "Herein does very much consist that image of God wherein He made man . . . viz in those faculties and principles of nature whereby he is capable of moral agency."[24] If Edwards was claiming that this capacity was unique to humans, then we have to ask how such a claim stands today in light of the developments in evolutionary psychology we reviewed earlier.

As we have seen, evolutionary psychologists are currently debating the significance of what appears to be altruistic behavior in animals. As some researchers suggest that nonhuman primates show primitive versions of a moral sense and moral agency, others remind us that we cannot really say what mechanisms—such as motivation, cognition, and willful agency—underlie behaviors that are only superficially similar.

For some evolutionary psychologists, the emergence of altruistic-looking behavior is explained by the almost mechanical and self-interested process called inclusive fitness (or "kin selection"), in which organisms aid close relatives to help their own genes survive. This behavior is extended to other organisms by "reciprocal altruism," a method of mutual survival. In this reciprocal theory, self-sacrifice is actually self-interest, expecting the other organism to repay the helpful deed in the future.

There has been considerable discussion as to whether reciprocal altruism and kin selection are really sufficient to explain human behavior.[25] A major problem is that humans cooperate in much larger groups than nonhuman primates, extending beyond those with whom they interact socially. Others have argued for "strong reciprocity" in humans. By this they mean a predisposition to cooperate with others and to punish those who don't cooperate, even though they suspect that they may not be repaid by others, even at a later date.[26] More controversially, sociobiologist David Sloan Wilson has broadened the idea of altruism between nonrelatives to a model of "group selection," which rivals the individual-selection model of orthodox Darwinian theory.[27]

Behavior that looks altruistic does not require self-awareness, as the behavior of insects or birds clearly illustrates. Based on this obvious fact, the evolutionary biologist Francisco Ayala rejects the idea that human ethical behavior arises simply from evolved social behavior in animals. The key measure for human altruism, he says, is the self-aware capacity for ethics: an ability to anticipate the results of one's actions, make value judgments, and choose between possible courses of action. This capacity to choose is basic to human nature, while the specific moral norms that guide actions are created by human culture and society over time. As Ayala explains, the capacity for ethics is a necessary and unique feature of being human. Arriving at particular moral norms is a secondary consequence, based on intellectual ability.[28]

THE NEW CONSENSUS ON *IMAGO DEI*

The contemporary theologian J. Wentzel van Huyssteen has traced the intellectual history of ideas about the *imago dei* and found three kinds of interpretation, as we saw earlier. These are the substantive, functional, and relational viewpoints.[29] Substantive interpretations identify a single property of each individual, such as reason, rationality, or intellect. These substantive interpretations have been dominant in the history of Western Christianity and thus, up until Aquinas, all Christian writers saw the image of God as humankind's power of reason. The functionalist view of the *imago dei* has been seen variously as exercising dominion and fulfilling stewardship of the creation. The relational view posits that humans bear the image of God in both the capacity for relationship and in the existence of a unique form of relationship between God and humankind.

After this long history of debate, the theological consensus is that the *imago dei* cannot be based singly on human anatomy, genes, neurology, or behavior. Instead, the image of God in humankind arises from a combination of structural, functional, and relational elements.[30] The consensus has also discounted the idea that the Genesis account (2:7) of the creation implies that a literal soul was breathed into the human body: "The Lord God formed a human being of the dust of the ground, breathed into his nostrils the breath of life, and the human being became a living soul." As the Bible scholar Joel Green points out, the term *soul* is used in Genesis for both humans and animals:

> The same term ("a living soul") is used only a few verses earlier with reference to "every beast of the earth," "every bird of the air" and "every thing that creeps on the earth"—that is, to everything in which there is life, demonstrating incontrovertibly that "soul" is not, under this accounting, a unique characteristic of the human person.[31]

Without recourse to a nonmaterial soul, religious believers are easily tempted to define what makes us uniquely human in terms of some specific human capacity and then to identify that with the *imago dei*. However, research comparing such capacities in humans and primates significantly reduces the credibility of such views. On the other hand, what seems to be a moral sense, moral agency, self-giving, or self-sacrifice in animals tells us nothing about the mechanisms and thinking patterns that underlie those behaviors. Self-giving behavior may, for example, occur with or without self-awareness.

Anthropologists can produce models of the descent of humanity that are self-contained and intellectually satisfying. Such models seldom conflict with the biblical record in any obvious way. This does not prove that God was or was not involved in the process. In the end, we believe that it is faith (*a priori* commitments), not sight (or scientific discovery) that convinces us of ultimate realities that we not see. By commitment, or by faith, we might "understand that the universe was formed by God's command, so that the visible came forth from the invisible" (Heb. 11:1, 3). In a scientific age, the challenge for the believer is to recognize God's divine upholding of the overall visible process.

With respect to human nature, we believe that the idea of God's image implies relationship and not any characteristic that would have left a mark in the paleoanthropological record. Beyond this, it is prudent to recall Donald MacKay's wise words that, as he put it, "with regard to those aspects of human nature that concern the scientist, the biblical data are much more reticent than is commonly supposed."[32]

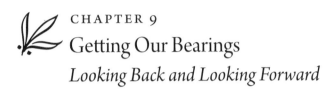

CHAPTER 9

Getting Our Bearings
Looking Back and Looking Forward

THE PAST HALF CENTURY has witnessed rapid, and some would say explosive, developments where psychology interfaces with neuroscience and with evolutionary biology. Research in neuropsychology has been greatly facilitated and accelerated by remarkable developments in brain-scanning methods. These rapid advances are reminiscent of developments in the first half of the twentieth century in evolutionary biology and in the second half of the twentieth century in genetics. In both cases, research findings challenged previously held beliefs about human nature and our place in the great scheme of things. Humanists and religious people each found some of their cherished beliefs called into question.

In each new era of research, the leaders invariably were both believers and atheists. The believers saw the science as explaining natural phenomena in a way that gave fresh insights into how God had created and continues to do so; the atheists saw the science as explaining away religion and emptying religious beliefs of meaningful content. One goal of this book is to survey the past encounters between science and religion in regard to psychology and brain science and to bring them up to date. Throughout, we have tried to draw wisdom and lessons from the excitement, false steps, and debates over the attempts of science and religion to answer the question posed by St. Augustine in his *Confessions*, book XI: "What am I?"

This history provides us with examples to follow as well as errors to avoid. In our time, we have seen a revival of the ideas of Sigmund Freud that belief in God is nothing more than a comforting illusion. This is evidenced by British biologist Richard Dawkins' popular book, *The God Delusion*. Furthermore, the rapid developments in cognitive neuroscience reminded us of the excitement caused by phrenology in the nineteenth century. Today, we are finding more and more correlations between religious behavior and brain processes. Just as phrenology looked to bumps on the head, we are looking at colorful images of blood flow in specific brain areas. As noted, this can be good science but also an invitation to unwarranted claims or speculation.

Fifty years into the "cognitive revolution," we are still asking questions that arose in centuries past: How do we define the "soul" today? Does this parallel the way we now talk about the mind? What does this say about the fundamental nature of human beings? Are we an aggregate of different parts glued together in some ill-defined way—a soul stuck to a body or to a brain—or are we a psychosomatic unity? In his work, *The Astonishing Hypothesis*, Francis Crick recognized that raising issues of this kind would present fundamental challenges to some religious beliefs deeply held for centuries and still widely held today. In the West, the belief endures that we have an immaterial immortal soul that is somehow and somewhere attached to our body. Many Christians believe that this is what the Bible teaches. However, as we noted, leading biblical scholars are opening the way for believers to hold a different "embodied" interpretation of the soul. In this book, we have argued that, by taking a new view of the soul, there is no necessary conflict between a biblical portrait of human nature, which emphasizes the unity of the human person, and a neuropsychological view of the relationship of mind and brain.

We have also noted, especially in our survey of phrenology, that there is a variety of possible ways to describe relationships between science and one's religious faith. For example, neuroscience can easily slip into an unthinking reductionism, in which human experience is "nothing but" a movement of molecules or chemicals. We also saw how it is possible for the over-enthusiastic nonscientist, assailed with today's dramatic brain-scanning images, to claim they prove we are locating a "spot" for every conceivable human activity—much as was done with the bumps of phrenology. These modern findings have been used by atheists to explain away the supernatural as merely an evolved capacity, but also by some religious persons who may want to show, using the research in "neurotheology," that a "God spot" in our brain proves that God exists.

In contrast to some of these extremes, we have tried to present a more holistic and complex view of the brain and human nature. In this model, our highest level and most sophisticated mental processes are fully embodied in our brains as formed by human culture. These brain-dependent processes allow for the emergence of personhood, as well as the evident richness of human society and culture, which, in turn, via social and developmental learning, influences the brain's networks of functional connections. It is no longer helpful or reasonable to consider the mind a nonmaterial Cartesian entity that can be decoupled from the body and the world. It is out of the continual experiences of behavior and environmental-societal feedback that the mind becomes formed as a functional aspect of our brain and body.

As a better alternative, we have espoused an *emergentist* view, which goes under several labels. Our preferred labels are either *non-reductive physicalism* or *dual-aspect monism*. Both labels underline the fact that, although humans are entirely physical beings, we cannot reduce all causes of human behavior to simple chemistry and physics. *Nonreductive* in the term *nonreductive physicalism* suggests this rejection of reducing all life to its simplest parts. Many "causes" in life lie in the emergent properties of the whole person. Our second preferred term, *dual-aspect monism*, singles out neither the physical nor the mental aspect of the whole of our mysterious nature, but says both aspects—the physical and the mental—are necessary to do justice to reality.

Whichever term we use, the mental side of our reality is paramount because that allows us to reflect on these matters in the first place! Thomas Nagel, a contemporary philosopher who writes on this topic, tells us that "so far as we can tell, our mental lives and those of other creatures, including subjective experiences, are strongly connected with and perhaps strictly dependent on physical events in our brains and on the physical interaction of our bodies with the rest of the physical world." Equally, Nagel has no doubts that "we have to reject conceptual reduction of the mental to the physical." But if that is the case, how are we to think about our mental world? He acknowledges that "the mind-body problem is difficult enough so that we should be suspicious of attempts to solve it with the concepts and methods developed to account for very different kinds of things. Instead we should expect theoretical progress in this area to require a major conceptual revolution." Nagel believes this will require a change in our thinking at least as radical as relativity theory was in physics. [1]

As we have seen, the new evolutionary psychology, like neuroscience, is presenting fresh challenges to traditional beliefs about human nature. Most recently, the scientific work in this field has sought the evolutionary origins of such seemingly distinctive human capacities as language, social relatedness, moral behavior, and altruism. But, as Frans de Waal has written in his work *Good Natured*, "direct comparisons between people and animals are often seen as demeaning, even offensive." Nevertheless, de Waal sees the results of research in evolutionary psychology not as demeaning, but rather as underlining the evolutionary origins of such behavior in, as he put it, "our much maligned human nature."

Evolutionary psychologists have no doubt that we can learn more about human evolution by studying the behavior of other animals and that, by this method, we may detect the possible beginnings of such human capacities as language, theory of mind, and culture in chimpanzees societies. They are equally clear, however, that we must be careful in extrapolating implications for human behavior from observations of other animals. Extrapolation is only justified if the scientific evidence warrants it. For example, a 2007 report in the journal *Science* reports empirical research that demonstrates that, while humans are "self-interested rational maximizers" in economic decision making, they also "take into account the interests of others and are sensitive to norms of cooperation and fairness." Our closest living phylogenetic relatives, the chimpanzees, are not sensitive to fairness, however. The researchers conclude, "These results support the hypothesis that other-regarding preferences and aversion to inequitable outcomes, which play key roles in human social organization, distinguish us from our closest living relatives."[2]

Each animal phylum is unique. Each has properties and abilities that none others do. Regarding humankind, however, evolutionary psychology has no interest in the *kind* of theological questions that are raised in the domain of Christian anthropology, which deals with the assertion that humans are called into a personal relationship with God. Evolutionary psychology has no views on such questions. Individual psychologists certainly have their personal beliefs on such issues, but those must be distinguished from the science itself.

Because some of our readers might be concerned about the apparent narrowing gap between ourselves and some nonhuman primates, it is important to reiterate that we do not see any great issues at stake here for the Christian. Careful workers in the field are themselves often dismayed by the use made of their findings in the media. A Christian can remain enthusiastically open-minded about developments in evolutionary psychology—not gullible, but discerning—and through this openness, glimpse fresh pointers to the greatness of the Creator and the wonders of his creation, of which we ourselves are a part.

Perhaps most disconcerting to religious persons has been the research on the relationship between brain activity and religious experiences. As we have seen, questions about important dimensions of human experience are raised by research into the relationship between religion and specific parts of the brain. These research findings include the link between religious experiences and some forms of temporal lobe epilepsy; the possibility of creating such experiences by magnetic stimulation of the brain or by imbibing certain hallucinogenic substances; and the neuroimaging studies showing that there may be a unique brain area or pattern of brain activation associated with religious experiences. However, here again, further reflection suggests that these scientific studies merely point to our "creatureliness" and the embodiment of our mental and religious experiences. They say nothing with respect to whether these experiences, when they occur, are linked to a reality outside of our selves. These studies merely demonstrate that our most meaningful and deeply personal experiences emerge from, and take place within, our physical selves.

Spirituality: Embedded and Embodied

So, what about "spirituality"? Cambridge University theologian Sarah Coakley has helpfully reminded us that "spirituality" has become a buzz word whose meaning often does not go beyond mere "hand waving."[3] Thus, it is important that anyone using the word be clear about its meaning. She points out that much "spirituality" is a controlled religious "high" that is devoid of the content normally necessary for the "spirituality" of Christian churchgoers: namely, the content of clear doctrinal beliefs. That more nebulous spiritual high also excludes people who see spirituality as living out a worldview in which the world, moment by moment, is upheld by a creator God.

Spiritual experiences may well be a social and cultural variable that guides our interpretations of certain forms of neural events. In other words, neurons are not creating our religions, but it's the other way around (our religions interpret our neuronal experiences). We have asked, for example: "Would the same neural events be considered religious by a participant if that person had no religious background whatsoever, or was not currently in a context that semantically primed religious interpretations?" People in a religious context are far more likely to interpret a brain event as a "spiritual" experience. As Christians, we believe religion and spirituality are engendered by our embeddedness in Christian community and all the activities that that entails, and not inner properties of the brain.

We assume that spirituality involves experience, belief, and action: experience, in terms of our awareness of the transcendent; beliefs, in terms of what we believe about God, about ourselves, and about the world in which we live; and action, in terms of how we live our lives. The research repeatedly highlights the intimate interdependence between brain processes, cognitive processes, and behavior and is relevant to understanding how those aspects of spirituality are mobilized and depend upon cognitive processes. Our experience is not free-floating and nonphysical, but firmly *embodied*. Such embodied beliefs and expectations are major factors in understanding some of the dimensions of life we might call "spiritual." At the same time, we recognize that cognitive processes such as beliefs and expectations are frequently held within social contexts, and that reminds us that spirituality is also firmly *embedded* within cultures and communities.

This perspective on the spiritual dimensions of life allows us to see broad realities. In one of them, the bottom-up approaches of neuroscience give special insights into understanding how changes in the neural structures of the brain manifest themselves in the subjective awareness and the objective expression of the religious life. In the second reality, top-down effects might give clues to how beliefs and expectations influence our physical health, such as the placebo effect (feeling better after taking a pill that really has no medical ingredient). In other words, the spiritual dimensions of our lives are *both* firmly *embodied* and *embedded*. As *embodied*, these dimensions are not immune to the effects of changes in the brain. As *embedded*, these religious dimensions of experience, belief, and practice also sculpt our brains and can bring about scientifically observed benefits such as optimism, health, and contentment.

We can be confident that spirituality is firmly embodied in our biological make-up. But that also means that the discussion about "the neurology of religion" is really only a convenient label, or shorthand, for talking about our basic neurological and cognitive capacities, which happen to underlie our special religious behaviors and experiences as well as many other human perceptions. The religious nature of these events results from personal beliefs and behaviors in social contexts. It is to these social contexts that we now turn as we consider the *embeddedness* of spirituality.

Except in very rare instances (such as the proverbial lonely hermit), the spiritual dimensions to life are lived out in community. As with all other aspects of our daily existence, our spirituality develops, is maintained, and manifests itself within community. It is fully embedded in our physical, cultural, and social environments. Embeddedness becomes important when, for example, discussing the spiritual dimensions of healing for which there is a substantial body of social and psychological research, extending over many decades, linking both personal and group beliefs with physical well-being.

In conclusion, we suggest that a helpful way to think about the relationship between the mental and physical aspects of our life is one of irreducible intrinsic interdependence that manifests duality without dualism. That is, the mental (and spiritual) are nested in, and dependent upon, our bodily systems. And yet, mental events demand a different level of both subjective and objective description.

While some of the research findings trumpeted by the popular media are indeed dramatic, they also raise new questions and demand better interpretations. Modern neuroscience is very much a "work in progress." We are watching a lively debate among scientific leaders at the cutting edge of the research, as well as one among philosophers, on how best to make sense of it all. There are no simple or easy answers.

Our human lives, with our beliefs and hopes, are both embodied in our physical brains and embedded in our societies and cultures, whether we as individuals happen to be religious are not. Our scientific understanding of human nature is advancing rapidly. In all likelihood, science will begin to decipher the operation of some of our most cherished religious experiences, such as sudden or "miraculous" conversions or healings. Religious beliefs, in general, and Christian faith in particular, must prepare for that day.

We believe that, for the future, the Christian emphasis on a moment-by-moment upholding of all creation by God is important. Such a view recognizes the spiritual dimensions of life as embodied and embedded. It also affirms that the whole of reality—all that we observe and are privileged to study—is a manifestation of the unchanging and steadfast love of a Creator who upholds all things at all times.

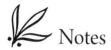 Notes

CHAPTER 1: NEUROSCIENCE AND PSYCHOLOGY TODAY

1. Fyodor Dostoyevsky, *The Idiot*, trans. Henry and Olga Carlisle (New York: Signet Classic, 1969), 245.
2. EU report on "Meeting of Minds" project, Jan. 23, 2006, at www.meetingmindseurope.org.
3. Howard M. Feinstein, *Becoming William James* (Ithaca, NY: Cornell University Press, 1984), 313.
4. H. Gardner, "Scientific Psychology: Should We Bury It or Praise It?" *New Ideas in Psychology* 10, no. 2 (1992):180.
5. Ibid.
6. R. Hooykaas, *Philosophia Libera: Christian Faith and the Freedom of Science* (London: Tyndale, 1957).
7. Malcolm A. Jeeves and R. J. Berry, *Science, Life, and Christian Belief* (Leicester, UK: InterVarsity Press and Baker, 1998).

CHAPTER 2: WARFARE VERSUS PARTNERSHIP

1. Laurence Hearnshaw, *A Short History of British Psychology* (London: Methuen, 1964).
2. Bronislaw Malinowski, *Sex and Repression in Primitive Society* (New York: Harcourt, Brace & Co., 1927); and *The Foundations of Faith and Morals* (London: Oxford University Press, 1936).
3. G. S. Spinks, *Psychology and Religion* (London: Methuen, 1963), 102.
4. B. F. Skinner, *Beyond Freedom and Dignity* (New York: Knopf, 1971), 116.
5. Roger W. Sperry, "Psychology's Mentalistic Paradigm and the Religion/Science Tension," *American Psychologist* 43, no. 8 (1988): 607–8.
6. Gordon W. Allport, *The Individual and His Religion: A Psychological Interpretation* (London: Constable, 1951), viii.
7. Frederic C. Bartlett, *Religion as Experience, Belief and Action* (Oxford: Oxford University Press, 1950), 4.
8. Hendrika Vande Kemp, "The Sorcerer as a Straw Man—Apologetics Gone Awry: A Reaction to Foster and Leadbetter 2," *Journal of Psychology and Theology* 15, no. 1 (1987): 20.

9. Richard Dawkins, *The God Delusion* (London: Bantam Press, 2007), as quoted by Robin Marantz Henig in "Darwin's God," *New York Times*, March 4, 2007, 2 (http://www.nytimes.com/2007/03/04/magazine/04evolution.t.html?page wanted=1&sq=Justin%20Barrett&st=nyt&scp=10.

10. William James, *The Varieties of Religious Experience* (London: Longmans, Green, and Co., 1902), as quoted in Henig, "Darwin's God," 2.

11. Stephen Jay Gould, *Rocks of Ages* (New York: Ballantine, 1999), as quoted in Henig, "Darwin's God," 5.

12. Justin Barrett, *Why Would Anyone Believe in God?* (Lanham, MD: Rowman Altamira, 2004), as quoted in Henig, "Darwin's God," 5, 13.

13. Francis Crick, *The Astonishing Hypothesis: The Scientific Search for the Soul* (New York: Touchstone, 1994), 621.

14. Roger W. Sperry, "Forebrain Commissures and Conscious Awareness," *Journal of Medicine and Philosophy*, 2, no. 2 (1977): 121.

CHAPTER 3: FROM SOUL TO MIND

1. Jean Baptiste Bouillaud, "Recherches cliniques propres à démontrer que la perte de la parole correspond à la lésion des lobules antérieurs du cerveau et à confirmer l'opinion de M. Gall, sur le siège de l'organe du langage articule" *Archives of Generales de Medecine* 8, 25–45.

2. François Gall and J. C. Spurzheim, *On the functions of the Brain and of Each of Its Parts: with Observations on the Possibility of Determining the Instincts, Propensities, and Talents, or the Moral and Intellectual Dispositions of Men and Animals, by the Configuration of the Brain and Head*, trans. Winslow Lewis, Jr. (Boston: Marsh, Capen and Lyon, 1835), 1:55.

3. Robert M. Young, *Mind, Brain and Adaptation in the Nineteenth Century: Cerebral Localization and Its Biological Context from Gall to Ferrier* (Oxford: Oxford University Press, 1990), 39, 43.

4. Quoted in ibid., 44.

5. Alfred R. Wallace, *My Life: A Record of Events and Opinions* (London: Chapman and Hall, 1905), 1:234–36.

6. Young, *Mind, Brain and Adaptation*, 44.

7. Franz Joseph Gall, *Des disposition innees* (Paris: Schoell, 1811), 292.

8. Robert W. Rieber, "The Multiplicity of the Brain, the Unity of the Soul and the Duality of the Mind: Can You Have It All the Way?," presentation given at the International Society for the History of the Neurosciences, Providence, RI, June 12, 2003.

9. Gall, *Des disposition innees*, 47.

10. Rieber, "Multiplicity of the Brain," 16.

11. Johann Casper Spurzheim, *A View of the Philosophical Principles of Phrenology*, 3rd ed. (London: Charles Knight, 1840), 100–108.

12. Wayne Norman and Malcolm A. Jeeves, "Neurotheology: The New Phrenology?," paper in preparation.

13. Scot W. Easton, *The Harmony of Phrenology with Scripture on the Doctrine of the Soul* (Edinburgh: Printed for the Author [by Dr. R. Collie & Son], 1867), 33.

14. William Scott, *The Harmony of Phrenology with Scripture* (Edinburgh: Fraser & Co., 1844), 178.

15. Carol Albright and James Ashbrook, *Where God Lives in the Human Brain* (Naperville, IL: Sourcebooks, 2001), 164.

16. Julia C. Keller, "Brushes with Death Transform Life and the Brain," *Science and Theology News*, (June 2004): 8.

17. Interview of Osamu Muramoto, "Cortex Keeps Time in the Brain's Religious Orchestra," *Science and Theology News*, 14, no. 10 (June 2004): 9.

18. Christopher Stawski, "Spiritual Transformation Q&A: Mario Beauregard," published online in *The Global Spiral* 4, no. 3 (March 1, 2004): 4. www.metanexus.net/Magazine/

19. Jerome Groopman, "God on the Brain," *The New Yorker*, September 17, 2001, 165.

20. Franz Joseph Gall, "Schreiben über seinen bereits geendigten Prodromus über die Verrichtungen des Gehirns der Menschen und der Thiere am Herrn Jos Fr von Retzer" *Der neue Teutsche Merkur*, 1798, 3:330, as cited in John van Wyhe, "The Authority of Human Nature: The *Schädellehre* of Franz Joseph Gall," *British Journal for the History of Science* 35, no. 124 (2002): 26.

Chapter 4: Principles of Brain Function

1. Preliminary figures courtesy of Michael L. Spezio and coworkers, Scripps College and Caltech. Research was funded by a grant from the Mind and Life Institute.

2. Gerald M. Edelman and Giulio Tononi, *A Universe of Consciousness: How Matter Becomes Imagination* (New York: Basic Books, 2000), 103.

Chapter 5: Linking Mind and Brain

1. David Hubel and Torsten Wiesel, "Receptive Fields, Binocular Interaction and Functional Architecture of the Cat's Visual Cortex," *Journal of Physiology* 160, no. 1 (1962): 106–54.

2. William Beecher Scoville and Brenda Milner, "Loss of Recent Memory after Bilateral Hippocampal Lesions," *Journal of Neurology, Neurosurgery and Psychiatry* 20, no. 1 (1957): 11–21.

3. R. W. Sperry, "Psychology's Mentalistic Paradigm and the Religion/Science Tension," *American Psychologist* 43, no. 8 (1988): 609.

4. Ibid., 607.

5. W. S. McCulloch and H. W. Garol, "Cortical Origin and Distribution of Corpus Callosum and Anterior Commissure in the Monkey (Macaca mulatta)," *J. Neurophysiol.* 4, no. 6 (1941): 555–63 as quoted in Philip Winn, *Dictionary of Biological Psychology* (London: Taylor and Francis, 2001), 185.

6. R. W. Sperry, "The Great Cerebral Commissure," *Scientific American* 210 (January 1964): 42–53.

7. Melissa Bateson, Daniel Nettle, and Gilbert Roberts, "Cues of Being Watched Enhance Cooperation in a Real-World Setting," *Biol Lett.* 2, no. 3 (2006): 412–14.

8. Rechele Brooks and Andrew N. Meltzoff, "The Importance of Eyes: How Infants Interpret Adult Looking Behavior," *Dev Psychol.* 38, no. 6 (2002): 958–66.

9. D. I. Perrett et al., "Neurons Responsive to Faces in the Temporal Cortex:

Studies of Functional Organisation, Sensitivity to Identity and Relation to Perception," *Human Neurobiology* 3, no. 4 (1984): 197–208.

10. K. M. O'Craven and N. Kanwisher, "Mental Imagery of Faces and Places Activates Corresponding Stimulus–specific Brain Regions," *Journal of Cognitive Neuroscience* 12, no. 6 (2000): 1013–23.

11. Nancy Kanwisher and Galit Yovel, "The Fusiform Face Area: A Cortical Region Specialised for the Perception of Faces," *Philosophical Transactions of the Royal Society of London B*, 361 (2006): 2123.

12. Christian Keysers and David Perrett, "Demystifying Social Cognition: A Hebbian Perspective," *Trends in Cognitive Sciences* 8, no. 11 (2004): 501–7.

13. Jeffrey M. Burns and Russell H. Swerdlow, "Right Orbitofrontal Tumor with Pedophilia Symptom and Constructional Apraxia Sign," *Archives of Neurology* 60, no. 3 (2003): 437.

14. Daniel T. Tranel, quoted by Chris Kahn in "Pedophile 'Cured' After Surgery," reported by the Associated Press, July 28, 2003.

15. Frans de Waal, *Good Natured: The Origin of Right and Wrong in Humans and Other Animals* (Cambridge, MA: Harvard University Press, 1997), 216–17.

16. T. W. Robbins et al. "Cognitive Deficits in Progressive Supranuclear Palsy, Parkinson's Disease, and Multiple System Atrophy in Tests Sensitive to Frontal Lobe Dysfunction," *J Neurol Neurosurg Psychiatry* 57, no. 1 (1994): 79–88.

17. Philip Winn, "Frontal Syndrome as a Consequence of Lesions in the Pedunculopontine Tegmental Nucleus: A Short Theoretical Review," *Brain Research Bulletin* 47, no. 6 (1998): 559.

18. C. Bernard Gensch et al. "Influence of Supplementary Vitamins, Minerals and Essential Fatty Acids on the Antisocial Behaviour of Young Adult Prisoners," *British Journal of Psychiatry* 181, no. 1 (2002): 22–28.

CHAPTER 6: THE HUMAN ANIMAL

1. See the entry for Lloyd C. Morgan in *The Oxford Companion to the Mind*, ed. Richard L. Gregory (Oxford: Oxford University Press, 1987), 496.

2. Jerome H. Barkow, Leda Cosmides, and John Tooby, eds. *The Adapted Mind: Evolutionary Psychology and the Generation of Culture* (New York: Oxford University Press, 1992), 7.

3. R. W. Byrne, "Evolutionary Psychology and Sociobiology: Prospects and Dangers," in *Human Nature*, ed. M. A. Jeeves, (Edinburgh: The Royal Society of Edinburgh, 2006) 84–105.

4. Frans De Waal, *Good Natured: The Origin of Right and Wrong in Humans and Other Animals* (Cambridge, MA: Harvard University Press, 1996), 64.

5. Amy S. Pollick and Frans B. de Waal, "Ape Gestures and Language Evolution," *Proc Natl Acad Sci USA* 104, no. 19 (2007): 8184–89.

6. T. J. Crow, ed., *The Speciation of Modern Homo Sapiens* (Oxford: Oxford University Press, 2003).

7. D. Premack and G. Woodruff, "Does the Chimpanzee Have a Theory of Mind," *Behavioral and Brain Sciences* 1, no. 4 (1979): 515–26.

8. Andrew Whiten and Richard Byrne, *Machiavellian Intelligence II: Extensions and Evaluations* (Cambridge: Cambridge University Press, 1997), 150.

9. Richard Byrne and Andrew Whiten, eds., *Machiavellian Intelligence: Social Expertise and the Evolution of Intellect in Monkeys, Apes and Humans* (Oxford: Clarendon Press, 1988).

10. Byrne, "Evolutionary Psychology and Sociobiology," 91.

11. Michael Tomasello, "Primate Cognition: Introduction to the Issue," *Cognitive Science* 24, no. 3 (2000): 357.

12. Michael Tomasello, Josep Call, and Brian Hare, "Chimpanzees Understand Psychological States—The Question Is Which Ones and to What Extent," *Trends in Cognitive Science* 7, no. 4 (2003): 153.

13. Simon Baron-Cohen, "I Cannot Tell a Lie," *In Character* 3, no. 3 (Spring 2007): 55–56.

14. Ibid., 56.

15. Giacomo Rizzolatti et al., "Premotor Cortex and the Recognition of Motor Actions," *Brain Res Cogn Brain Res* 3, no. 2 (1996): 131–41.

16. Vittorio Gallese, "Before and Below 'Theory of Mind': Embodied Simulation and the Neural Correlates of Social Cognition," *Philos Trans R Soc Lond B Biol Sci* 362, no. 1480 (2007): 659–69.

17. V. S. Ramachandran, interview with Tom Stafford, *The Psychologist* 17, no. 11 (November 2004): 636–37.

18. Andrew Whiten, "The Place of 'Deep Social Mind' in the Evolution of Human Nature," in *Human Nature*, ed. M. Jeeves (Edinburgh: The Royal Society of Edinburgh, 2006), 212.

19. Byrne, "Evolutionary Psychology and Sociobiology," 99.

20. John M. Allman et al., "Intuition and Autism: A Possible Role for Von Economo Neurons," *Trends Cogn Sci* 9, no. 8 (2005): 367–73.

21. John M. Allman et al., "The Anterior Cingulate Cortex: The Evolution of an Interface between Emotion and Cognition, *Ann NY Acad Sci* 935 (2001): 107–17.

22. Esther A. Nimchinsky et al., "A Neuronal Morphologic Type Unique to Humans and Great Apes," *Proc Natl Acad Sci USA* 96, no. 9 (1999): 5268–73.

23. de Waal, *Good Natured*, 12.

24. Ibid., 208.

25. Ibid., 218.

26. Byrne, "Evolutionary Psychology and Sociobiology," 96.

27. Blaise Pascal, *Pensees*, trans. Roger Ariew (Indianapolis: Hackett Publishing, 2005), 33.

28. John Polkinghorne, *The Way the World Is* (London: SPCK, 1983), 55.

Chapter 7: The Neuroscience of Religiousness

1. David E. Nichols and Benjamin R. Chemel, "The Neuropharmacology of Religious Experience: Hallucinogens and the Experience of the Divine," in *Where God and Science Meet: Volume Three, The Psychology of Religious Experience*, ed. Patrick McNamara (Westport, CT: Praeger, 2006), 1–34.

2. Ibid., 26.

3. Ibid., 3.

4. Haruhiko Naito and Nozomi Matsui, "Temporal Lobe Epilepsy with Ictal

Ecstatic State and Interictal Behavior of Hypergraphia," *Journal of Nervous and Mental Disease* 176, no. 2 (1988): 123–24.

5. V. S. Ramachandran et al., "The Neural Basis of Religious Experiences," *Society for Neuroscience Conference Abstracts* (1997): 1316.

6. J. L. Saver and J. Rabin, "The Neural Substrates of Religious Experience," *Journal of Neuropsychiatry* 9, no. 3 (1997): 498.

7. See Michael A. Persinger and Katherine Makarec, "Temporal Lobe Epileptic Signs and Correlative Behaviors Displayed by Normal Populations," *Journal of General Psychology* 114, no. 2 (1987): 179–95; and Michael A. Persinger and Katherine Makarec, "Complex Partial Epileptic Signs as a Continuum from Normals to Epileptics: Normative Data and Clinical Populations," *Journal of Clinical Psychology* 49, no. 1 (1993): 33–45.

8. Pehr Granqvist et al., "Sensed Presence and Mystical Experiences Are Predicted by Suggestibility, Not by the Application of Transcranial Weak Complex Magnetic Fields," *Neuroscience Letters* 379, no. 1 (April 29, 2005): 1–6.

9. A. Newberg et al., "The Measurement of Regional Cerebral Blood Flow during the Complex Cognitive Task of Meditation: A Preliminary SPECT Study," *Psychiatry Research: Neuroimaging*, 61, no. 2 (2001): 113–22.

10. Preliminary data from Spezio and colleagues, op. cit.

11. N. P. Azari et al., "Neural Correlates of Religious Experience," *European Journal of Neuroscience* 13, no. 8 (2001): 1649–52.

12. A. Newberg et al., "The Measurement of Regional Cerebral Blood Flow during Glossolalia: A Preliminary Study,"*Psychiatry Research: Neuroimaging* 148, no. 1 (2006): 67–71.

13. This research is reviewed in Lindon Eaves, "Genetic and Social Influences on Religion and Values" in *From Cells to Souls—and Beyond: Changing Portraits of Human Nature,* ed. Malcolm Jeeves (Grand Rapids, MI: Eerdmans, 2004), 102–22.

14. This argument comparing religion and baseball is also made in Warren S. Brown, "The Brain, Religion, and Baseball: Comments on the Potential for a Neurology of Religion," In *Where God and Science Meet: How Brain and Evolutionary Studies Alter Our Understanding of Religion; Volume II: The Neurology of Religious Experience,* ed. Patrick McNamara, (Westport, CT: Greenwood Press, 2006) 229–44.

15. These two studies are described in J. D. Greene et al., "The Neural Bases of Cognitive Conflict and Control in Moral Judgment," *Neuron* 44, no. 2 (2004): 389–400; and in J. D. Greene et al., "An fMRI Investigation of Emotional Engagement in Moral Judgment," *Science* 293, no. 5537 (2001): 2105–8.

16. For current analyses of Capgras syndrome, see N. M. Edelstyn and F. Oyebode, "A Review of the Phenomenology and Cognitive Neuropsychological Origins of the Capgras Syndrome," *International Journal of Geriatric Psychiatry* 14 (Jan. 1999): 48–59; W. Hirstein and V. S. Ramachandran, "Capgras Syndrome: A Novel Probe for Understanding the Neural Representation of the Identity and Familiarity of Persons," *Proceedings of the Royal Society of London. Series B: Biological Sciences* 264 (March 1997): 437–44; and M. J. Mentis et al., "Abnormal Brain Glucose Metabolism in the Delusional Misidentification Syndromes: A Positron Emission Tomography Study in Alzheimer Disease" *Biological Psychiatry* 38 (Oct. 1995): 438–49.

17. Simon Baron-Cohen, Alan M. Leslie, and Uta Frith, "Does the Autistic Child Have a 'Theory of Mind'?" *Cognition* 21, no. 1 (1985): 37–46.
18. Fulvia Castelli et al., "Autism, Asperger's Syndrome and Brain Mechanisms for the Attribution of Mental States to Animated Shapes," *Brain* 125, no. 8 (2002): 1839–49.
19. Alan G. Sanfey et al., "The Neural Basis of Economic Decision-Making in the Ultimatium Game," *Science* 300, no. 5626 (2003): 1755–58.
20. Brooks King-Casas et al., "Getting to Know You: Reputation and Trust in a Two-Person Economic Exchange," *Science* 308, no. 5718 (2005): 78–83.
21. Naomi I. Eisenberger, Matthew D. Lieberman, and Kipling D. Williams, "Does Rejection Hurt? An fMRI Study of Social Exclusion," *Science* 302, no. 5643 (2003): 290–92.
22. Tania Singer et al., "Empathy for Pain Involves the Affective But Not Sensory Components of Pain," *Science* 303, no. 5661 (2004): 1157–62.
23. Wolfhart Pannenberg, *Systematic Theology*, vol. 2 (Grand Rapids, MI: Eerdmans, 1944), 182; as quoted by Joel Green, "What Does It Mean to Be Human?" in *From Cells to Souls—and Beyond*, ed. Jeeves, 180.

CHAPTER 8: SCIENCE, RELIGION, AND HUMAN NATURE

1. Donald M. MacKay, *Human Science and Human Dignity* (Downers Grove, IL: InterVarsity Press, 1979), 27.
2. John C. Eccles, *Evolution and the Brain: Creation of the Self* (London: Routledge, 1989), 327.
3. Gerald M. Edelman, *Bright Air, Brilliant Fire: On the Matter of the Mind* (London: Penguin, 1982), 113.
4. R. W. Sperry, "Consciousness and Casuality" *The Oxford Companion to the Mind*, ed. Richard L. Gregory (Oxford: Oxford University Press, 1987), 165.
5. Roger Penrose, *The Emperor's New Mind* (Oxford: Oxford University Press, 1989), 580.
6. Nancey Murphy, "Nonreductive Physicalism: Philosophical Issues," in *Whatever Happened to the Soul? Scientific and Theological Portraits of Human Nature*, ed. Warren S. Brown, Nancey Murphy, and H. Newton Malony, (Minneapolis, MN: Fortress Press, 1998) 127–48. Also see Nancey Murphy and Warren S. Brown, *Did My Neurons Make Me Do It? Philosophical and Neurobiological Perspectives on Moral Responsibility and Free Will* (Oxford: Oxford University Press, 2007).
7. This section draws heavily on the work of Alicia Juarrero, *Dynamics in Action* (Chicago: Bradford Books, 1999); and on Murphy and Brown, *Did My Neurons Make Me Do It?*
8. Gerald M. Edelman and Giulio Tononi, *A Universe of Consciousness: How Matter Becomes Imagination* (New York: Basic Books, 2000), 211.
9. Alison Brooks, "What Is a Human? Archaeological Perspectives on the Origins of Humanness," in *What Is Our Real Knowledge of the Human Being*, Scripta Varia 109 (Vatican City: Pontificia Academia Scientiarum, 2007), 35.
10. Quotations in this paragraph come from ibid., 35.
11. Editorial, "Nature and the Brain," *Nature* 447 (June 14, 2007), 753.

12. Andrew Whiten, "The Place of 'Deep Social Mind' in the Evolution of Human Nature," *Human Nature*, ed. M. A. Jeeves (Edinburgh: The Royal Society of Edinburgh, 2006), 207.

13. Ibid.

14. Walter Bodmer, "Foreword," in *What Makes Us Human*, ed. Charles Pasternak (London: One World, in press).

15. Catechism of the Catholic Church, part 1, sec.1, chap. 1, sub-sec. 3, paragraph 36 (see http://www.vatican.va/archive/ENG0015/__PB.HTM). Modifications of this catechism were formally promulgated in the edition typical of the Catechism of the Catholic Church in September 1997 by Pope John Paul II.

16. Colin Gunton, *The Promise of Trinitarian Theology*, 2nd ed. (Edinburgh: T. & T. Clark, 1997), 101.

17. Kate Arnold and Klaus Zuberbühler, "Semantic Combinations in Primate Calls," *Nature* 441 (May 18, 2006): 303. See also Sue Savage-Rumbagh, Stuart G. Shanker, and Talbot J. Taylor, *Apes, Language and the Human Mind* (New York: Oxford University Press, 1998).

18. Joshua M. Plotnik, Frans B. M. De Waal, and Diana Reiss, "Self-recognition in an Asian Elephant," *Proceedings of the National Academy of Sciences of the US* 103, no. 45 (2006): 17055.

19. Frans de Waal, *Bonobo: The Forgotten Ape* (Berkeley: University of California Press, 1997).

20. Gerhard von Rad, *Genesis: A Commentary*, trans. J. H. Mark (London: SCM Press, 1972).

21. Warren S. Brown, "Cognitive Contributions to Soul," in *Whatever Happened to the Soul? Scientific and Theological Portraits of Human Nature*, eds. Warren S. Brown, Nancey Murphy, and H. Newton Malony (Minneapolis, MN: Fortress Press, 1998), 99–126.

22. Claus Westermann, *Genesis 1–11*, trans. J. J. Scullion (London: SPCK, 1984), 158.

23. Claus Westermann, *The Genesis Accounts of Creation*, trans. N. E. Wagner (Philadelphia: Fortress, 1964), 21.

24. Jonathan Edwards, "On the Freedom of the Will," part 1, sec. 5, *Concerning the Notion of Liberty, and of Moral Agency*; as referenced in George Marsden, *Jonathan Edwards* (New Haven, CT: Yale University Press, 2002).

25. Philip Clayton and Jeffrey Schloss, eds., *Evolution and Ethics* (Grand Rapids, MI: Eerdmans, 2004).

26. H. Gintis et al., "Explaining Altruistic Behaviour in Humans," *Evolution and Human Behavior* 24, no. 3 (2003): 153–72.

27. David Sloan Wilson, *Darwin's Cathedral* (Chicago: University of Chicago Press, 2003).

28. Francisco J. Ayala, "Human Nature: One Evolutionist's View," in *Whatever Happened to the Soul?* ed. Brown, Murphy, and Malony, 31–48.

29. J. Wentzel van Huyssteen, *Alone in the World? Human Uniqueness in Science and Theology* (Grand Rapids, MI: Eerdmans, 2006).

30. J. Richard Middleton, *The Liberating Image: The Imago Dei in Genesis 1* (Grand Rapids, MI: Brazos Press, 2005).

31. Joel B. Green, "What Does It Mean to Be Human?" In *From Cells to Souls—and Beyond*, ed. M. A. Jeeves, (Grand Rapids, MI: Eerdmans, 2004), 196.

32. Donald M. MacKay, *Brains, Machines and Persons* (London: Collins; Grand Rapids, MI: Eerdmans, 1980), 48.

CHAPTER 9: GETTING OUR BEARINGS

1. Thomas Nagel, "Science and the Mind-Body Problem," in *What Is Our Real Knowledge about the Human Being* (Vatican City: Pontifica Academia Scientiarum, 2007), 96, 99, 100.

2. Keith Jensen, Josep Call, and Michael Tomasello, "Chimpanzees Are Rational Maximizers in an Ultimatum Game," *Science* 318, no. 5847 (2007): 107–9.

3. Sarah Coakley, "Spiritual Healing: Science, Meaning, and Discernment," in *Introduction to Spiritual Healing in a Post-Modern Age: Scientific Explanation, Cultural Diversity, and the Problem of Meaning,* ed. Sarah Coakley (Grand Rapids, MI: Eerdmans, in preparation).

Further Reading

Albright, Carol, and James Ashbrook. *Where God Lives in the Human Brain.* Naperville, IL: Sourcebooks, 2001.

Allport, Gordon W. *The Individual and His Religion: A Psychological Interpretation.* London: Constable, 1951.

Bartlett, Frederic C. *Religion as Experience, Belief and Action.* Oxford: Oxford University Press, 1950.

Brown, Warren S., Nancey Murphy, and Newton H. Malony, eds. *Whatever Happened to the Soul? Scientific and Theological Portraits of Human Nature.* Minneapolis: Fortress Press, 1998.

Byrne, Richard W., and Andrew Whiten, eds. *Machiavellian Intelligence: Social Expertise and the Evolution of Intellect in Monkeys, Apes and Humans.* Oxford: Clarendon Press, 1988.

Clayton, Philip, and Jeffery Schloss, eds. *Evolution and Ethics.* Grand Rapids, MI: Eerdmans, 2004.

Crick, Francis. *Astonishing Hypothesis: The Scientific Search for the Soul.* New York: Touchstone, 1994.

Damasio, Antonio. *Descartes' Error: Emotion, Reason, and the Human Brain.* New York: Penguin Putnam, 1994.

Dawkins, Richard. *The God Delusion.* London: Bantam Press, 2006.

Dennett, Daniel C. *Elbow Room: The Varieties of Free Will Worth Wanting.* Cambridge, MA: Bradford Books, 1984.

de Waal, Frans. *Bonobo: The Forgotten Ape.* Berkeley: University of California Press, 1997.

———. *Good Natured: The Origin of Right and Wrong in Humans and Other Animals.* Cambridge, MA: Harvard University Press, 1997.

Edelman, Gerald M. *Bright Air, Brilliant Fire: On the Matter of the Mind.* London: Penguin, 1982.

Edelman, Gerald M., and Giulio Tononi. *A Universe of Consciousness: How Matter Becomes Imagination.* New York: Basic Books, 2000.

Flanagan, Owen. *The Problem of the Soul: Two Visions of Mind and How to Reconcile Them.* New York: Basic Books, 2002.

Fuster, Joquín M. *Cortex and Mind: Unifying Cognition.* Oxford: Oxford University Press, 2003.

Gallese, Vittorio. "Before and Below 'Theory of Mind': Embodied Simulation and the Neural Correlates of Social Cognition." *Philos Trans R Soc Lond B Biol Sci,* 362, no. 1480 (2007): 659–69.

Gould, Stephen Jay. *Rocks of Ages: Science and Religion in the Fullness of Life.* New York: Ballantine, 1999.

Hofstadter, Douglas. *I Am a Strange Loop.* New York: Basic Books, 2007.

James, William. *The Varieties of Religious Experience.* London: Longmans, Green, and Co., 1902.

Jeeves, Malcolm A., ed. *From Cells to Souls—and Beyond: Changing Portraits of Human Nature.* Grand Rapids, MI: Eerdmans, 2004.

———., ed. *Human Nature.* Edinburgh: The Royal Society of Edinburgh, 2006.

Jeeves, Malcolm A., and R. J. Berry. *Science, Life, and Christian Belief.* Leicester, UK: Intervarsity Press and Baker: 1997.

Juarrero, Alicia. *Dynamics in Action.* Chicago: Bradford Books, 1999.

MacKay, Donald M. *Behind the Eye: The Gifford Lectures.* Edited by Valerie MacKay. Oxford: Basil Blackwell, 1991.

———. *Brains, Machines and Persons.* London: Collins and Grand Rapids, MI: Eerdmans, 1980.

———. *Human Science and Human Dignity.* Downers Grove, IL: InterVarsity Press, 1979.

McNamara, Patrick, ed. *Where God and Science Meet: How Brain and Evolutionary Studies Alter Our Understanding of Religion.* 3 vols. Westport, CT: Greenwood Press, 2006.

Murphy, Nancey. *Bodies and Souls, or Spirited Bodies?* New York: Cambridge University Press, 2006.

Murphy, Nancey, and Warren S. Brown. *Did My Neurons Make Me Do It? Philosophical and Neurobiological Perspectives on Moral Responsibility and Free Will.* Oxford: Oxford University Press, 2007.

Pasternak, Charles, ed. *What Makes Us Human.* London: One World, 2008.

Penrose, Roger. *The Emperor's New Mind.* Oxford: Oxford University Press, 1989.

Polkinghorne, John. *The Way the World Is.* London: SPCK, 1983.

Quartz, Steven R., and Terrence J. Sejnowski, *Liars, Lovers, and Heroes: What the New Brain Science Reveals About How We Become Who We Are.* New York: HarperCollins, 2002.

Russell, Robert John, Nancey Murphy, Theo C Meyering, and Michael A Arbib, eds. *Neuroscience and the Person*. Notre Dame, IN: University of Notre Dame Press, 2000.

Salzman, Mark. *Lying Awake*. New York: Alfred A. Knopf, 2000.

Savage-Rumbaugh, Sue, and Roger Levin. *Kanzi: The Ape at the Brink of the Human Mind*. New York: John Wiley & Sons, 1994.

Skinner, B. F. *Beyond Freedom and Dignity*. New York, Knopf: 1971.

Sperry, Roger W. *Science and Moral Priority: Merging Mind, Brain, and Human Values*. New York: Columbia University Press, 1983.

Spinks, G. S. *Psychology and Religion*. London: Methuen, 1963.

Thouless, Robert H. *An Introduction to the Psychology of Religion*. 1923. 3rd ed. London: Cambridge University Press, 1971.

Van Huyssteen, J. Wentzel. *Alone in the World? Human Uniqueness in Science and Theology*. Grand Rapids, MI: Eerdmans, 2006.

Whiten, Andrew and Richard W. Byrne. *Machiavellian Intelligence II: Extensions and Evaluations* Cambridge: Cambridge University Press, 1997.

Wilson, David Sloan. *Darwin's Cathedral*. Chicago: University of Chicago Press, 2003.

Young, Robert M. *Mind, Brain and Adaptation in the Nineteenth Century: Cerebral Localization and Its Biological Context from Gall to Ferrier*. Oxford: Oxford University Press, 1970.

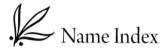

Name Index

Subject Index